Vision and Brain

Vision and Brain

How We Perceive the World

James V. Stone

The MIT Press
Cambridge, Massachusetts
London, England

MIT Press books may be purchased at special quantity discounts for business or sales promotional use. For information, please e-mail special_sales@mitpress.mit.edu or write to Special Sales Department, The MIT Press, 55 Hayward Street, Cambridge, MA 02142.

This book was set in Stone Sans and Stone Serif by Toppan Best-set Premedia Limited, Hong Kong. Printed and bound in the United States of America.

Library of Congress Cataloging-in-Publication Data

Stone, James V., Dr.
Vision and brain : how we perceive the world / James V. Stone.
    p. cm.
Includes bibliographical references and index.
ISBN 978-0-262-51773-7 (pbk. : alk. paper)
1. Visual perception. 2. Vision. I. Title.
BF241.S77 2012
152.14–dc23
2011052297

10 9 8 7 6 5 4 3 2 1

To Verity, Chris, Dorian, and Bob

Some may fear that such a materialistic outlook, which regards the brain as a kind of super machine, will take the magic out of life and deprive us of all spiritual values. This is about the same as fearing that a knowledge of human anatomy will prevent us from admiring the human form. Art students and medical students know that the opposite is true. The problem is with the words: if machine implies something with rivets and ratchets and gears, that does sound unromantic. But by machine I mean any object that does tasks in a way that is consonant with the laws of physics, an object that we can ultimately understand in the same way we understand a printing press. I believe the brain is such an object.

—David Hubel, *Eye, Brain, and Vision* (1988)

Philosophy is written in this grand book—the universe—which stands continuously open to our gaze. But the book cannot be understood unless one first learns to comprehend the language and interpret the characters in which it is written. It is written in the language of mathematics . . . without which it is humanly impossible to understand a single word of it; without these one is wandering about in a dark labyrinth.

—Galileo Galilei (1564–1642), *The Assayer*

Contents

Preface

This book tells the story of how we see. It is a story with only two characters, the physical world and the brain. The physical world is a cunning, deceitful character, full of lies, or worse, half-truths. It is not to be trusted at any time, nor at any cost. The brain is a flawed detective with a loaded die for a compass, working on lousy pay with fuzzy data, and a strict, sometimes literal, deadline. But over eons of evolutionary time, the brain has always had one crucial advantage: it knows that the physical world has to play by certain rules, rules that are ultimately derived from the laws of physics. Armed with this singular insight, the brain tests and retests, millisecond by millisecond, multiple competing hypotheses about what in the world might have produced the evidence of its own eyes, ruthlessly casting aside red herrings and fallguys one by one, by one, until there is only a single suspect who does not have a rock-solid alibi: and that is the one chosen by the brain, that is what we *see*.

Scientific Revolutionaries

If you really want to understand how science works then don't read this book. Read books written by scientists who were revolutionaries, scientists who simply stepped over the cutting edge of conventional science to create whole new fields of research. For physics, read Albert Einstein's *Relativity: The Special and the General Theory* (1920) or Richard Feynman's lectures (Feynman, Leighton, & Sands 1964); for evolution, read Charles Darwin's *On the Origin of Species* (1859); and for information theory, read Claude Shannon and Warren Weaver's *The Mathematical Theory of Communication* (1949). These are the scientists who defined whole new areas of investigation, scientists who created a new research field, and made it shine. Their books are beacons of insight and wisdom. More importantly, these books demonstrate how scientific skepticism can be used to ask the right questions, and how not to be fooled by the physical world, or by yourself (as Richard Feynman said, "The first principle is that you must not fool yourself, and you are the easiest person to fool").

Vision and Brain: How We Perceive the World is intended as a companion to John Frisby's and my more comprehensive book, *Seeing: The Computational Approach to Biological Vision* (2010). A small amount of the material in *Seeing* is inevitably duplicated here (after all, there's only one human visual system to describe).

The title of this book is a little ambiguous. The question implicit in the title is: "How does the brain see the world? At one level, the answer might be a description of how individual neurons react in response to particular retinal images. But this would be like asking how a video camera works and being told the changing voltages of every component inside the camera. In one sense, this is a complete answer, but it is essentially useless in terms of understanding how a video camera works. At a different level, the answer could consist of a description of which different brain regions seem to be activated by different visual features, such as color, motion, or faces. But this would be like being told which of the various electronic modules in the camera was responsible for each different function without being told how each module works. Admittedly, these two extreme scenarios are caricatures, but they do give an impression of the different approaches to understanding vision. Now supposing we assume that the brain, in contrast to a video camera, behaves according to a set of well-defined principles, principles that dominate its processing at every level within the system. One consequence of making this assumption is that it forces us to reformulate questions about vision and the brain in an increasingly rigorous and mathematically succinct manner. Armed with these questions, the answers obtained take the form of rigorous and transparent mathematical models. Even though the details of such models would normally demand some mathematical expertise, the principles on which they are based are, in essence, simple, and even obvious. *Vision and Brain* is intended to provide an account of these principles, the principles that seem to underpin how the brain sees the world, but without the distracting mathematical details that such rigor usually entails. Accordingly, this book provides an account of the principles on which vision and brain function may be based, but it requires that readers have only a high school level of mathematical competence. In writing what I hope is an accessible survey of modern findings on vision, I've been inspired by Marr's computational framework (1982), the efficient coding hypothesis (Atick & Redlich 1992; Attneave 1954; Barlow 1961; Laughlin 1981), Bayesian inference (Bayes 1763), and information theory (Shannon & Weaver 1949).

We begin with an overview of vision. This is followed by an examination of the particular nature of the problems faced by the brain in attempting to solve the problems of vision, but portrayed in the context of general principles that may allow it to do so. The all-too-thin line between accessibility and the larger (usually complicated) truth is trodden with some care, and when the occasional wobble leaves the reader on the wrong side of this line, reassurance is provided in the form of frequent informal summaries. This book is based on the philosophy that every key idea should be accompanied by an explanatory figure, and these figures should also help to keep the reader on the right side of that narrow line. And if the text appears overly simplistic in places, this is because there are no depths to which I will not sink (in terms of simplicity, diagrams, and analogies) in order to explain a complex idea to willing but inexpert readers. So, if you want to understand the scientific basis of human vision then read on.

Acknowledgments

Thanks to my wife and colleague, Nikki Hunkin, for all sorts of help and advice and to our children, Sebastian and Teleri, for helping to ensure that at least some of the ideas expressed here possess the simplicity demanded by the crystal-clear logic of a child's mind. Thanks to David Buckley for his enthusiasm for vision, to Pasha Parpia for long conversations on the nature of brain science, to John DePledge for making me think hard about Satosi Watanabe's ugly duckling theorem (which is why it was removed), to Steve Snow and also Royson Sellman for pointing out the limits of stereopsis and parallax, and to Chris Williams for comments on Bayes's theorem.

Several colleagues and friends have generously given up their time to read a draft of this book. I wish to express my gratitude in particular to David Buckley, Stephen Eglen, John Frisby, Nikki Hunkin, Stephen Isard, Pasha Parpia, and Tom Stafford. I hope that psychologists Buckley, Frisby, Hunkin, and Stafford find the mathematical ideas in this book clear, and I apologize to mathematician Isard, physicist Parpia, and computational biologist Eglen for bastardizing some beautiful theorems to force them through the word colander that an introductory textbook demands (and to SE for both).

Thanks to Bob Prior, Susan Buckley, Katherine Almeida and many others at MIT Press for advice in completing the various tasks involved in writing a book.

Finally, thanks to the University of Sheffield for standing by the noble tradition that a university has a duty to share the knowledge of its academics not only with students, but with the widest possible audience.

The Party Trick

It was a Christmas party in 2010, and I sat munching snacks. He just came up to me, shook my hand, and said hello. Then he took two rubber bands out of his pocket; he looped one over my thumb and forefinger and one over his, except that, together, our bands formed a one-link chain. And I realized that he and now I were part of the entertainment. Then he did something extraordinary. He moved his hand back, so that his link pulled my link toward him, and his rubber band simply *passed through* mine. Apparently, the link had been broken, except that both rubber bands were intact. He looked at me expectantly as the applause broke out. "Very impressive," I said, but my voice was a flat monotone. "'Wow' is the usual response," he said. "I teach vision," I said.

It took me a little time to work out why I said that. But, once I had, I wish I'd said this:

I teach vision, about how the brain manages to see the world, despite objects that hide among their own shadows, the lousy lens of the eye, the back-to-front photoreceptors, the cussed nature of rainbowed light, the blood vessels that run amok over the retina and shield photoreceptors from that light, the squelching of 126 million photoreceptors' information into the one million cables of the optic nerve, the transformation from a fuzzy photograph-like retinal image to a series of Morse code-like blips that race into the brain's recesses, where the retina's image is corrupted by the stark unreliability of neuronal components that are the shrapnel of the Cambrian explosion from 543 million years ago. We know a large number of facts, a virtual archipelago of clues, about how this machine works, but we do not understand why it works as well as it does. That it works at all seems little short of miraculous, and the more facts we gather about each part, the less we seem to understand about the whole, and the more miraculous it seems. So when you seem to pull your rubber band through mine, I know it's a trick, but my incomprehension is immeasurably trivial compared to the ancient arc of steely ignorance that shields us from the knowledge of how we manage to see any rubber band. That's the mystery. Not how my visual system can be tricked so that it sees something that could not possibly exist, but how any visual system, annealed in the unknowing cauldron of evolution, *sees anything*.

1 Vision: An Overview

And here we wander in illusions.
—William Shakespeare, *Macbeth*

Impressions

Photons smash into the eye's darkness, deforming light-sensitive molecules, causing a cascade of chemical fallout, ending only when a stream of spikes escapes through the backdoor of the eye. These are coded messages from the dazzling world. Unscrambled, they command pictures in the head, with spectral order, and a particular beauty. They burst un-bidden, from eyes that cannot themselves see, and shower the brain with information, until, in that dark place, these messages let there be light.

All that you see, all that you have seen, and everything you will ever see is delivered to your brain as a stream of digital pulses whizzing along the fragile threads of salty, fluid-filled cables that are your nerve fibers. These nerve fibers, or *neurons*, are the only connection between you and the physical world, and the pulses they deliver are the only messages you can ever receive about that world. Once the enormous implications of this fact are appreciated, it no longer seems remarkable that we can experience illusions and even hallucinations. Instead, what does seem remarkable is that anyone ever sees anything at all, or at least anything that actually exists.

How We See: The Brain as a Detective
Seeing is very easy—and very hard. Look around you: it is easy to see the world. Now try to explain how you see that world, and you will begin to find out how hard seeing really is. But you are in good company because the truth is that nobody knows exactly how we see, even though there is an enormous body of knowledge about optics, the eye, and the brain. This book is a brief account of that knowledge.

The brain is constantly doing its best to find out what in the world is responsible for the image on the retina. In essence, this is the central problem of vision. It's as if the brain is a detective at the scene of a murder, with the retinal image as the body. But this is a case that would defeat even the great Sherlock Holmes. There are many clues, but they're scattered over a large area. The suspects are many, but devious, and all of them have both motive and opportunity. But the worst of it is that all the suspects who don't have rock-solid alibis appear to be equally and utterly guilty. In the face of so much evidence, the brain, drawing on some 3.8 billion years of inherited evolutionary experience, does what it does best: it makes an intelligent guess. Its trick is to arrive at a guess as good as it can possibly be while taking into account every quantum of evidence and every iota of past experience—a guess that is *optimal*.

Illusions: How the Brain Fails?

We can find clues to how the brain works in the ways it fails to work when confronted with particular optical illusions. First, the brain has to find ways to see beyond the image in order to see what is probably in the world, by compensating for information *missing* from the retinal image, as shown in figures 1.1 and 1.2. Second, the brain has to see what is in the world by sometimes disregarding information that is *present* in the retinal image. For example, in order to see the patches on the cube in figure 1.3 (plate 1) as different shades of gray, the brain has to disregard the fact that they are the same shade of gray on the page. Let's briefly consider several illusions in terms of how the brain fails to work.

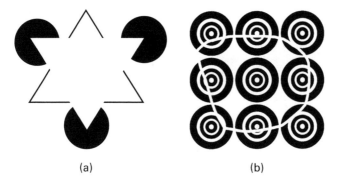

(a)   (b)

Figure 1.1
(a) Kanizsa triangles show that some lines are more apparent than real. (b) Variant on the Kanizsa illusion. The white curve is apparent, but not real, within and between the nine sets of concentric disks. Created by author.

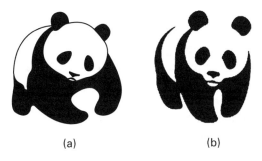

(a)   (b)

Figure 1.2
Disappearing lines of the World Wildlife Fund panda logo between 1961 (a) and 2006 (b). Lines around the head and back that are real in (a) are merely apparent in (b). Reproduced with permission.

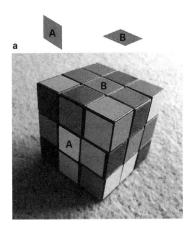

Figure 1.3 (plate 1)
Edited image of a Rubik's cube. The patch labeled A on the side of the cube and the red patch labeled B on the top of the cube share the same color on the printed page, as can be seen when they're shown isolated above the photograph. This illusion was created simply by copying the color of B to A using a graphics application. Based on an illusion by Ted Adelson. From Frisby & Stone 2010.

Illusory Lines: Triangles and Pandas

For the brain to see what's in the world rather than simply what's in a retinal image, it sometimes has to "fill in the gaps" in the image. Although doing this works in general, it can also result in optical illusions, such as in the Kanizsa triangles shown in figure 1.1a. At first glance, it is not obvious that this is an illusion at all: the picture simply seems to portray two overlapping triangles. On closer examination, however, it's apparent that one triangle has edges only within the cut-out regions of the black disks. The illusion is also supported by the gaps in the black lines, which suggest that something (i.e., another triangle) is covering up parts of the black lines. Together, these fool the brain into guessing that there are two overlapping triangles, even though there clearly are not. Surprisingly, the Kanizsa triangles do not disappear on ce the basis of the illusion is known. It is as if the visual system uses a self-contained logic of its own, which is immune to the knowledge that the triangles are illusory. Artists are well aware of the brain's ability to "fill in the gaps," as shown in figure 1.2 by the disappearing lines in the World Wildlife Fund logo between 1961 and 2006.

Recognizing Objects: Cubes, Rings, and Pianos

For the brain to see the three-dimensional structure of what is in the world, it has to ignore all but one of the possible 3-D structures that could have given rise to the retinal image. This is demonstrated in figure 1.4, where two different 3-D interpretations can be perceived. If you look at the star in the center of the figure, at one moment the rings appear to be viewed from above, but at the next moment they seem to be viewed from below. A more extreme example is shown in figure 1.5, where the shape in the retinal image (shown at the bottom) could have been formed by any one of the three 3-D objects shown above it. This, in turn, implies that any one of the 3-D objects shown would have generated *exactly the same* retinal image. How does the brain know which one?

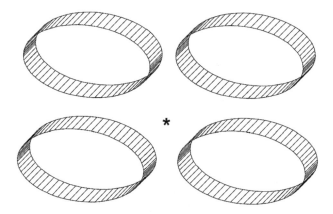

Figure 1.4
Look at the star in the center of the figure. At one moment, the rings appear to be viewed from above, but at the next moment they seem to viewed from below. Created by author.

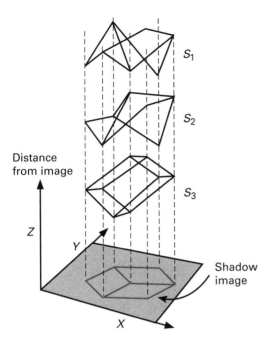

Figure 1.5
The fact that every retinal image could have been produced by many possible scenes is a major problem for the brain. Each of three different wire-frame objects yields exactly the same image (bottom). Adapted with permission from Kersten & Yuille 2003.

Fortunately, the brain can rely on its previous experience to exclude 3-D shapes only rarely encountered in the past. Because cubes are more common than all the other 3-D shapes that could have generated this retinal image, the brain is able to choose the cube as the single most probable 3-D interpretation of the inherently ambiguous shape on the retina.

This general rule of thumb, or *heuristic*, of excluding rare, and therefore improbable, 3-D interpretations is smarter than it might first appear. This is because the 3-D shapes shown in figure 1.5 are three examples from an infinite number of 3-D shapes, each of which would have generated the same the retinal image. Thus, by choosing a cube as the most probable 3-D shape, the brain effectively excludes an infinite number of other possible 3-D interpretations.

The ambiguity of retinal images has been used to good effect by artists such as Shigeo Fukuda, whose jumbled piano, shown in figure 1.6, is a compelling example. Here the piano seen in the background is actually the

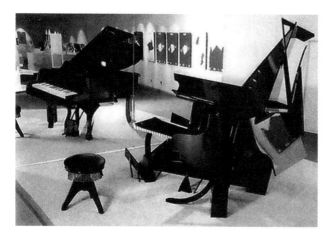

Figure 1.6
Piano or pile of wood? It all depends on your point of view. By Shigeo Fukuda.

reflection in a mirror of the jumble of wood shown in the foreground. In other words, if you were to stand where the mirror is then the jumble of wood would appear to be a piano. As with the example of a wire-frame cube, the image of a jumble of wood has an infinite number of possible 3-D interpretations (e.g., a 3-D jumble of wood). Moreover, all but one of these interpretations have probably never been seen before and are therefore rejected by the brain. In contrast, the single 3-D structure that is consistent with the retinal image is, of course, a piano.

Although these examples include 3-D objects deliberately designed to generate the required images, the general point remains: experience is required to disambiguate images. More importantly, using previous experience to interpret ambiguous retinal images can be made mathematically precise by making use of the *Bayesian framework*, a topic to which we will return in chapter 6.

Perceiving Three-Dimensional Shape: Shading, Craters, and Faces
The contours apparent in figure 1.7 (plate 2) are almost entirely based on the subtle changes in shading across the image, which is an important visual cue regarding the three-dimensional structure of a surface. Crucially, shading can be used to find a 3-D structure only if the viewer knows where the light source is in relation to the viewed scene. This becomes obvious if we trick the visual system into assuming the light is coming from the wrong direction. Thus both pictures in figure 1.8 depict the Barringer meteor crater in northern Arizona, except that one is upside down. But,

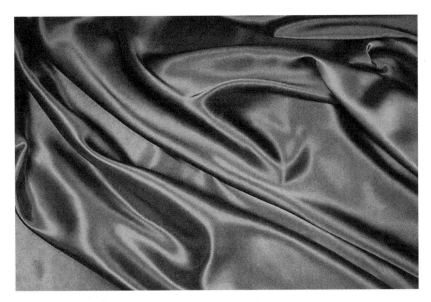

Figure 1.7 (plate 2)
Silk sheet. The three-dimensional shape perceived here is almost entirely due to subtle changes in shading.

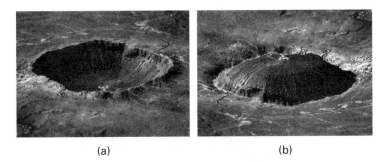

(a)   (b)

Figure 1.8
Are these pictures of a hill or a crater? It all depends on your point of view. Barringer Meteor Crater, reproduced with permission from the United States Geological Survey.

in both cases, the brain assumes that the light comes from *above*. This is true for figure 1.8a, which is therefore perceived as a crater. However, for figure 1.8b, this assumption forces the brain to perceive the crater as a hill (because a hill is all it could be if the light came from above). As with the example of wire-frame objects in figure 1.5, the brain is forced to interpret an image that is fundamentally ambiguous by adding its own bias. For figure 1.8b, this bias takes the form of an assumption about where the light source is likely to be, and a reasonable guess seems to be "from above."

Whether this "light-from-above" assumption is innate or based on previous experience is not known for sure. One of the first scientists to study this effect, David Brewster (1826), noted that children did not always interpret such pictures as if light came from above. More recently, it has been found that, as children grow older, they have an increasing tendency to perceive pictures like those in figure 1.8 as adults do (i.e., figure 1.8a as a crater and figure 1.8b as a hill; Thomas, Nardini, & Mareschal 2010; Stone & Pascalis 2010).

However, it is not hard to show that the assumption that light comes from above is more of a broad hint than an assumption that is rigidly applied to all images. When confronted by the image of a face defined almost entirely by changes in shading, as in figure 1.9, the brain appears willing to discard the light-from-above assumption, in favor of a more compelling assumption (more compelling in the context of faces, that is).

Figure 1.9 shows four frames from the movie of a rotating hollow mask, where the light comes from above. For the first three frames (a–c), the assumption that light comes from above leads to the perception of a convex (sticking-out) face. However, the fourth frame (d) shows the *concave* (hollow) inside of the mask, but it still appears to be *convex*.

When compared to the number of times normal (convex) faces are encountered, hollow faces are exceedingly rare. Consequently, the brain excludes the possibility that this could be a hollow face. But this choice

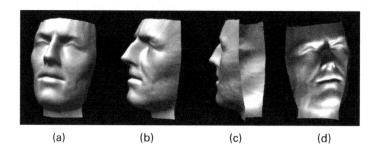

| (a) | (b) | (c) | (d) |

Figure 1.9
Face mask seen from four different positions with light coming from above. (a–c) Views from the front and sides create perceptions of a normal convex face. (d) View from the rear of the mask creates perception not of a concave face, as it "should" do, but again of a convex face. To achieve this incorrect perception, the brain is forced to assume that the light is coming from below. Courtesy Hiroshi Yoshida.

poses a dilemma. For the face in frame d to be seen as convex, the brain must assume that the light is coming from *below*. In other words, the image in figure 1.9d can be perceived either as a convex face with light from below or as a concave face with light from above. Self-evidently, the brain chooses the first interpretation because that's what we *see*. Indeed, the bias for seeing faces as convex is so strong that it is almost impossible for most adults to see frame d as a hollow face with light coming from above.

In short, it seems that the assumption that faces are convex effectively vetoes the assumption that light comes from above in the presence of images of faces. This, in turn, suggests that there may be a hierarchy of assumptions, with more important assumptions over-riding lesser assumptions in the interpretation of particular types of images. As we will see in chapter 6, these types of assumptions can be formalized within the Bayesian framework.

Shades of Gray and Grays of Shade

A piece of coal in bright sunshine reflects many times more light than a piece of white paper does in the relative darkness of a moonlit night. So why does the paper still appear as white and the coal as black? A clue to the answer can be gleaned from pictures such as the one in figure 1.10. Even though the upper surface is perceived as if it is darker than the lower surface, both surfaces have the same *albedo* (shade of gray) on the printed page.

The reason for this illusion is that the three-dimensional structure of the scene implies that the lower surface is in shadow, and that the upper surface is well lit. If this were the case for a 3-D object then the only way for the upper and lower surfaces to have the same gray level on the page (and therefore in the retinal image) would be if the upper surface were darker than the lower surface *on the object*. So this illusion has a rational basis in terms of the 3-D scene depicted. Again, the brain manages to see beyond the image on the retina to the underlying lightness of surfaces in the world. Moreover, it is precisely this ability to see past the retinal image that gives rise to the illusion depicted here.

Color and Shade

Look again at figure 1.7 (plate 2). The silk material does not change color, even though the changing three-dimensional contours of the silk sheet ensure that the image is darker or lighter in different places. The brain has managed to correctly interpret these image changes as changes in surface orientation rather than changes in the color of the material itself. Here the

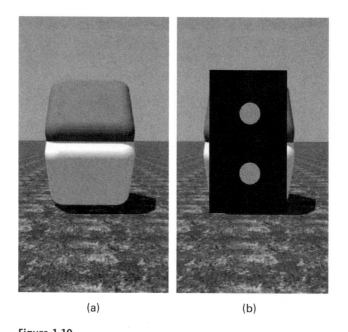

(a)   (b)

Figure 1.10
Surfaces in shadow are perceived as being lighter. (a) Both the upper and lower surfaces have the same albedo (shade of gray) on the page, which can be seen in (b), where a black card with holes has been placed in front of the object. The illusion of unequal lightness on the page seen in (a) is due to the fact that the upper surface is in the light whereas the lower surface is in shadow on the three-dimensional object. Reproduced with permission.

(less than obvious) illusion is that we see a constant color across the silk sheet, despite the changing shade of red across the image.

The converse of this is shown in figure 1.3 (plate 1). Here two patches of color on different sides of a Rubik's cube yield identical patches of color on the printed page, which are nevertheless perceived as different colors on the three-dimensional object. As we have already seen with figure 1.10, this can be explained by the shadow that falls over the patch on the side of the cube. Thus, the brain seems to reason, if both patches have the same color in the image and one of them is in shadow on the object then the shadowed patch must be lighter on the object. Notice that, to perceive this illusion, the brain must first work out the 3-D structure of the scene portrayed; otherwise, the two patches are perceived to be the same color (can be seen by viewing the patches in isolation, as in the top part of figure 1.3b).

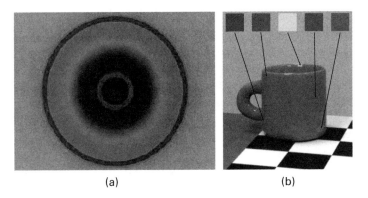

(a)   (b)

Figure 1.11 (plate 3)
Color illusions. A single color at two different locations on the page gives rise to the perception of two different colors in (a), whereas many different colors on the page give rise to the perception of a single color in the world in (b). The square patches at the top of the figure show the colors on the page from the locations indicated by the arrows. Reproduced with permission from (a) MacLeod (2003) and (b) Brainard & Maloney (2011).

Thus, in figure 1.7 (plate 2), the brain effectively ignores *changes* across the image in order to perceive the same color across the three-dimensional surface of the silk sheet. Conversely, in figure 1.3 (plate 1), the brain effectively ignores the *similarity* of colors of two patches in the image in order to perceive two different colors on the object's surface. A similar example of this can be seen in figure 1.11b (plate 3). In both cases, the brain takes account of the three-dimensional structure of the scene in order to interpret the colors depicted in the image.

Brains, Vision, and Bird Flight

Because human vision depends on neurons, it is tempting to think that all of the examples presented here can be explained in terms of the particular neuronal machinery of the brain. However, one of the revolutionaries of vision science, David Marr (1982, p. 27) famously used the analogy of flight to argue against studying *only* neurons in order to understand vision: "Trying to understand vision by studying only neurons is like trying to understand bird flight by studying only feathers: it just cannot be done."

Many of the early pioneers of human flight mistakenly believed that human flight should imitate bird flight in almost every detail. Accordingly, they built machines covered in feathers or machines with wings that flapped. In so doing, they mistook the particular trappings of how birds fly for the general principles of flight. For Marr, such principles emerge from a *computational analysis*, an analysis that considers not only how birds fly, but how flight can be achieved by any animal or machine, with or without feathers, with or without flapping. In other words, a computational analysis considers the *bare necessities* of attaining flight and the *principles* that *underpin* flight, without being constrained to copy the materials (feathers) and methods (flapping) used in any of the particular biological examples that exist in the natural world (e.g., birds).

In retrospect, it seems obvious that the Wright brothers' first powered flight in 1903 succeeded precisely because they took great pains to ensure that they understood the general principles of controlled flight (figure 1.12). More importantly, they understood that flight does not necessarily require feathers or flapping.

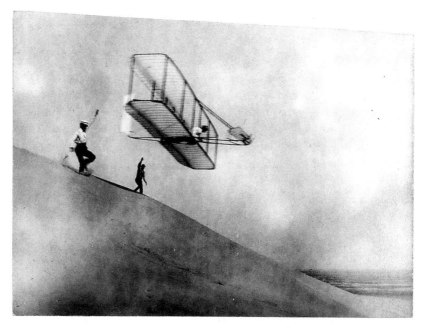

Figure 1.12
"Trying to understand vision by studying only neurons is like trying to understand bird flight by studying only feathers: it just cannot be done" (Marr 1982, p. 27). The Wright brothers were the first to successfully fly in 1903 because they understood the computational nature of the problem of flight, whereas many inventors insisted on mimicking the superficial aspects of flight (e.g., by building machines with flapping, feather-covered wings). This is a picture of the Wright brothers' 1902 glider.

Similarly, Marr argued that a proper understanding of the problem of vision can only be achieved by a full understanding of the computational principles on which vision is based. A computational analysis of vision considers the bare necessities of seeing and the principles of seeing, without being constrained to use the same materials (neurons) and methods (chemical messengers) used by the particular biological examples that exist in the natural world (brains). The abstract nature of Marr's computational framework is entirely compatible with recent developments in computational neuroscience, which suggest that the efficient coding hypothesis and information theory have much to offer the science of seeing; these ideas will be explored in subsequent chapters.

Marr's choice of the term *computational framework* is unfortunate, suggesting as it does that vision must function like a computer. Perhaps a more accessible term would be *informational framework* because Marr was keen to emphasize the nature of the information being processed without necessarily referring to the particular nature of the machinery (e.g., neurons or silicon chips) that happened to process that information. So, for Marr, it would matter little whether the device that is seeing was built from neurons, silicon, or wood, provided it sees and, more important, sees in the same way we do. But, you might ask, how could a device built from silicon see as we do?

We can explore this question by taking an extreme example from the realms of the philosophy of artificial intelligence. Quite simply, if one of the neurons in your brain were to be replaced with an electronic device that was, in every other respect, identical to that neuron, do you think you or the rest of your brain would notice? No. Now, suppose this was repeated, one by one, for all of the neurons in your brain. You would be, to all intents and purposes, the same person. Indeed, you would argue that you *are* the same person now as you were last year, even though many individual proteins in your brain have been replaced with (probably) identical ones. The point is that, as far as the *function* of each individual neuron is concerned, it does not matter what it is made of. Similarly, when it comes to considering how the brain performs the many tasks implicit in vision, it does not matter that it happens to be made of neurons. It does matter if we want to find out how a neuron helps solve the problems of vision, but it does not matter if we want to find out how any system, whether it is made of neurons or silicon, solves the problems of vision.

The above quotation from Marr was his protest against a purely reductionist approach, which would involve searching for the essence of vision only in the neuronal machinery of the brain. Thus, even though Marr did take account of findings from neurophysiology, he was also aware of the pitfalls of relying too heavily on such findings in order to understand vision. In essence, he proposed that, in formally describing how the brain solves the many problems implicit in vision, we should take account of neurophysiological, anatomical, and psychophysical data.

Because the following detailed discussion is fairly abstract, you may wish to return to it after first reading the remainder of the book. Marr's computational framework embodies three distinct, though not entirely independent, *levels of analysis*:

1 *Computational theory*   What is the nature of the problem to be solved, what is the goal of the computation, why is it appropriate, and what is the logic of the strategy by which it can be carried out?
2 *Representation and algorithm*   How can this computational theory be implemented? In particular, what is the representation for the input and output, and what is the algorithm (method) for transforming input to output?
3 *Hardware implementation*   How can the representation and algorithm be realized physically?

At the level of *computational theory*, the nature of the visual task to be solved should be formulated as precisely as possible. For example, this might entail finding the shape of three-dimensional objects from shading information. An *algorithm* is another word for a precise method. At this level, the amount of shading at each point in an image might be represented as a single number, and the local orientation of each corresponding point on the surface might be represented as a small plane (which requires two numbers to represent its orientation). The algorithm used to transform image gray levels into surface orientation could make use of the constraint that the local orientation of most objects varies smoothly from place to place on the object (although we would need more details to make such an algorithm work in practice). Finally, the *hardware implementation* could be executed using neurons, or a computer, for example.

Although each analytical level places constraints on the level below it, it does not *determine* its exact form. For example, the problem of obtaining shape from shading (see figure 1.7, plate 2) at the computational level specifies the nature of the problem for the algorithmic level, but this could be solved by a number of different algorithms at that level. Provided an algorithm solves the problem specified at the computational level, it doesn't matter which algorithm is used. In turn, each algorithm could be implemented at the hardware level by using either neurons or computers.

Again, provided a hardware implementation executes the specified algorithm, it doesn't matter which implementation is used. There is thus a cascade of influence, from the computational to the hardware level.

In reality, these levels are rarely independent of one another, and influences travel up and down between the levels. Moreover, it's difficult to find even one algorithm that solves a given computational problem and even one hardware implementation that executes the specified algorithm. In its defense, however, the computational framework forces the essential elements of any theory of vision to be specified with transparency and precision. This means that the strengths and flaws of a theory are easy to spot, which ensures that improvements to the theory are relatively easy to make. The computational framework is essentially both a recipe for how to study human vision, but it is also a recipe for how to study the human brain.

Unfortunately, Marr died (aged 35) before he could bring his work to fruition. But he left a rich legacy of ideas and a precise framework for how these ideas could be developed, ideas which have inspired subsequent generations of vision scientists.

Conclusion

The examples presented in this chapter are not only intriguing, they are also informative. They demonstrate that, to see the world as it is, the brain has to *interpret* the retinal image, which is full of lies and omissions. The brain's task is to see beyond these, to ignore the lies and fill in the omissions. Fortunately, the lies and omissions don't change from day to day but are law-like and systematic, and this systematicity allows the brain to correctly interpret all but the most ambiguous retinal images. Using Marr's framework to consider the problem of vision from a computational perspective, especially in the context of the efficient coding hypothesis and information theory, can inform us not only *how* the brain sees the world, but *why* the brain sees the world as it does.

2 Eyes

The eye, to this day, gives me a cold shudder.
—Charles Darwin

Impressions

The doors of perception through which we view the world were first opened as experiments in desperation. Out there, beyond the vista of our senses is a raging cacophony of interacting events, too fast and too slow, at frequencies too high and too low, to be detectable by us. These are the things that our evolutionary forebears, playing in the primordial casino, rejected as useless. Had they not done so, we might see colors beyond the limited spectrum now available to our eyes: infrared to see in the dark, ultraviolet to see through fog. We could track in slow motion the beat of a hummingbird's wing, and be distracted by the sudden unfurling of rose petals. Had they not done so . . .

The Evolution of Eyes

Even though life has existed on Earth for about 3.8 billion years, for some 3.3 billion of those years there were no eyes worthy of the name. When the first primitive eyes finally evolved early in the Cambrian explosion (around 543 million years ago; Land & Nilsson 2002), an arms race between the hunters and the hunted fueled the development of increasingly advanced visual systems. This would have forced prey to evolve camouflage coloration, and to remain still in the presence of predators, who then evolved color and stereo vision to penetrate that camouflage, and exquisitely sensitive motion detectors to detect any prey that dared to move. And here we are, the product of that arms race, able to track the tumbling flight of a fly, to hit a tennis ball in mid-flight, to spot red fruit on a background of green leaves, and to recognize each other from the subtle differences in our faces.

Darwin's Cold Shudder

The human eye is a complex structure, as shown in figure 2.1. How did such a structure evolve? This is a conundrum that exercised Charles Darwin, who was clearly tempted to throw up his hands in despair. "The eye, to this day, gives me a cold shudder," he wrote botanist Asa Gray in 1860, "but when I think of the fine known gradation, my reason tells me I ought to conquer the cold shudder."

Despite his own misgivings at an intuitive level, Darwin (1859) did not permit unfettered intuition to get in the way of logical reasoning:

If numerous gradations from a perfect and complex eye to one very imperfect and simple, each grade being useful to its possessor, can be shown to exist; if further, the eye does vary ever so slightly, and the variations be inherited, which is certainly the case; and if any variation or modification in the organ be ever useful to an animal under changing conditions of life then the difficulty of believing that a perfect and complex eye could be formed by natural selection, though insuperable by our imagination, can hardly be considered real.

The logic in this rather convoluted quotation has been supported by empirical comparative studies of eye design across different species, as well as by mathematical analyses that suggest a simple eye could have evolved over 400,000 generations (Nilsson & Pelger 1994), along the lines shown

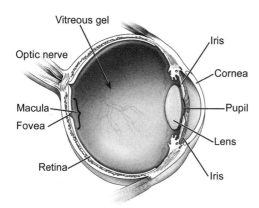

Figure 2.1
Human eye is essentially like a camera. Reproduced courtesy of National Eye Institute, National Institutes of Health.

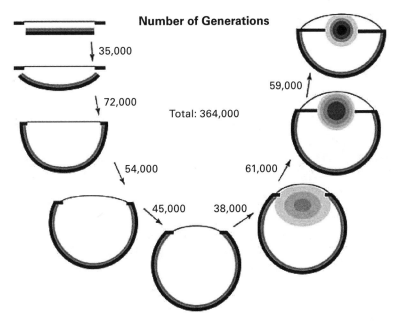

Figure 2.2
Evolution of the eye from a layer of light-sensitive cells to a fully formed imaging system. Based on a model proposed by Dane Nilsson and Susanne Pelger (1994), the number next to each figure indicates the number of generations required to make the transition from one stage to the next. Reproduced with permission.

in figure 2.2. This may sound like a long time, but if each generation lasted one year then the eye could have evolved in less than half a million years or, if each generation lasted ten years, in about 5 million years. Either way, such apparently large numbers represent little more than the blink of an eye when compared to the 3.8 billion years that life has existed on Earth.

The Simplest Eyes

The simplest type of "eye" is a globule of light-sensitive material suspended inside a single-celled organism like the *Euglena*, shown in figure 2.3. *Euglena* is part animal and part plant. Like an animal, it can move, using its whip-like tail to pull itself through the water, and it eats by enveloping food particles. Like a plant, it contains many *chloroplasts*, each of which uses sunlight to photosynthesize sugar; if *Euglena* can get itself to a place where there's light thenit can benefit from the sugars produced by its chloro-plasts. The *Euglena*'s eye is probably the oldest type of animal eye because

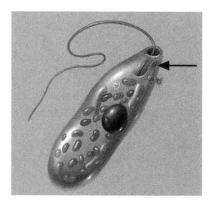

Figure 2.3
Drawing of a microscopic single-celled plant-animal (*Euglena*) showing an eye spot (arrow) next to the *flagellum* (whiplike structure) at its anterior (front). Reproduced with permission.

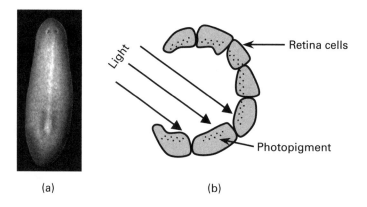

(a)   (b)

Figure 2.4
(a) Flatworm planarium has primitive black eyespots (this planarium is about 2 mm in length). Courtesy Creative Commons. (b) Cup-shaped, lensless eye of a planaria shown in cross section. Planaria can be found on the underside of rocks in streams. (b) by Sebastian Stone.

protists (the group of organisms to which *Euglena* belongs) are thought to have evolved about 2 billion years ago.

Within multicellular organisms, the eye can be as simple as a cup-shaped indentation of light-sensitive cells, as in the planaria (figure 2.4). The cup shape is important because it ensures that light coming from one

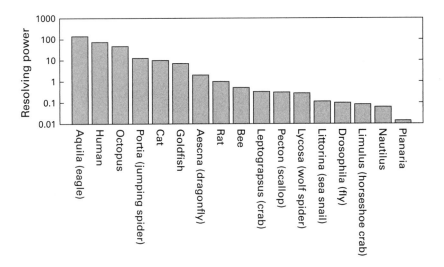

Figure 2.5
Comparative resolving power of eyes in different species, measured in cycles per degree. The logarithmic vertical axis, while allowing the enormous range to be included, masks the fact that the eagle (140 cycles per degree) can see about twice as well as a human (73 cycles per degree). Data replotted from Land 2002.

direction stimulates cells on only one side of the retina. Planaria can use this differential activation to determine where the light's coming from and therefore which way to go to seek refuge. This is obviously useful, but still leaves the planaria's eye at the bottom of the league of animal eyes (figure 2.5).

The Simple Eye

We have what's called a "simple eye." For our purposes, a *simple eye* is one that can form an image on the back of the eye or *retina* with or without a lens. This design is shared by all vertebrates (e.g., mammals, reptiles, and fish), squid and octopuses, jumping spiders, and an ancient group of species called "ammonites," which have only one living relative, the *Nautilus*. The fact that the simple eye is possessed by animals in such diverse phyla suggests that it has evolved independently many times (Land & Nilsson 2002).

A simple eye, like most cameras, has a lens but, again like a camera, it can also work without one. To understand how it does this, let's consider the simplest camera of all.

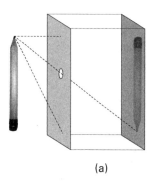 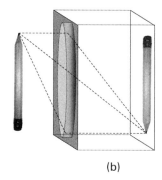

(a)   (b)

Figure 2.6
(a) Pinhole optics. Only those light rays bouncing off an object which happen to pass through the pinhole contribute to the image, which is therefore quite dim. Because these rays can travel only in straight lines from the object to the image, the image is upside-down and left-right reversed. (b) Lens ensures that many light rays from each point on the object converge on a single point in the image, yielding a bright image.

The Pinhole Camera

The image at the back of a pinhole camera (figure 2.6a) is always in focus, provided the pinhole is sufficiently small. (If the hole is too small then the wave characteristics of light take the form of diffraction artifacts, but we'll ignore these here.) The pinhole at the front of the camera ensures that each point in the image at the back of the camera receives light from only a single point in a scene, hence the camera's perfect focus. But the price paid for this perfect focus is that the image is dim because a pinhole doesn't let in much light. An obvious solution would be to make the hole bigger. That would make the image brighter—but also blurrier: by allowing light rays from each point in a scene to contribute to a larger region in the image, a larger pinhole effectively "smears" every point in the scene across the image.

The *Nautilus*'s eye is essentially a spherical pinhole camera (see figure 2.7) 10 millimeters (1 centimeter) in diameter, except that *Nautilus*'s pinhole or *pupil* can vary between 0.4 mm and 2.8 mm, depending on the amount of ambient light (Land & Nilsson 2002). Like the pinhole of our simplest camera, if the pupil is made small then the image is sharp but dim, whereas if it's made large, then the image is bright but blurred. *Nautilus* is a creature trapped between two visual worlds: one that is bright but too blurred to see any detail, and the other that is sharply focused but too dim to see anything much at all. This may explain why its eye comes pretty

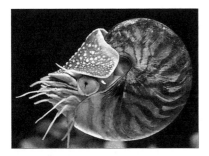

Figure 2.7
Nautilus, showing the large "pinhole" in a lensless eye. Reproduced with permission from Jochen Maes.

near the bottom of the league of animal eyes (figure 2.5). Indeed, it's remarkable that this animal has managed to survive for some 500 million years, longer than most species on Earth, with such a poor (though clearly adequate) eye.

If, however, all the rays passing through the pupil from a single point in the scene could be made to converge to a single point in the image then the image would not only be bright; it would also be in focus. The device that achieves this is the *lens*, as shown in figure 2.6b. Evidence that eyes with lenses aren't difficult to evolve is implicit in the sheer number of animal groups that have independently evolved them, including most cephalopods (e.g., squid, cuttlefish, but not *Nautilus*), fish, gastropods (e.g., snails and slugs), and arthropods (e.g., crabs and spiders).

The Human Eye

The human eye, shown in figure 2.1, is 24 millimeters in diameter, about the size of a golf ball. The outermost layer of the eye is the *conjunctiva*. The small chamber formed between the transparent *cornea* and the colored *iris* is filled with a fluid or *aqueous humor*, and the eyeball itself is filled with a jellylike fluid or *vitreous humor*. Just like a modern camera, the human eye has an adjustable circular aperture, the pupil, controlled by a ring of muscles within the iris.

Whereas a camera focuses the image by moving the lens back and forth, the human eye does so by altering the shape of the lens. The lens is quite flexible: it would adopt a spherical shape but for the constant tension from ligaments that pull on it, flattening its profile. The flatter lens focuses objects at far distances. When the ring of *ciliary muscles* that surround it contract, however, the tension on the lens is reduced, allowing it to relax into a more spherical shape, which brings nearby objects into focus. In fact, most of the focusing power of the eye depends on the fixed shape of the *cornea*. The lens simply fine-tunes the focus of the image on the retina.

If the lens is flexible then the eye's method for focusing the image works well. When, however, the lens becomes rigid with age, reducing the eye's ability to focus over a range of distances, we need different glasses to focus at different distances. In contrast, a fish eye focuses the image in the same way a camera does, by moving the lens back and forth, which may explain why even a 205-year-old rougheye rockfish (*Sebastes aleutianus*), landed off Newfoundland, was perfectly happy not to be wearing spectacles.

An Organ of Imperfections

Darwin referred to the eye as "an organ of extreme perfection," and, as we've already seen, it troubled him how such a thing could be the product of natural selection. Yet, though the eye is undeniably a remarkable structure, it's far from perfect. Among the eye's worst faults are chromatic aberration and optical imperfections, which cause image distortions, and the fact that the photoreceptors point the wrong way (toward the *back* of the eye).

Chromatic aberration is the blurring of an image caused by the inability of the lens to focus light of all different colors on the retina at the same time. In figure 2.8 (plate 4), light from part of a hat contains a mixture of yellow and blue colors. As light passes through the lens, its path is bent, but the amount of bending depends on the color of the light, with red being bent least, blue being bent most, and yellow light being bent somewhere in between. This means that when the lens is adjusted to focus all of the light of one specific color on the retina, the light of any other color remains out of focus, and thus forms a fuzzy image on the retina. Because the eye is most sensitive to red and green light—a mixture that looks yellow— yellow is the color of light brought to a focus on the retina in figure 2.8 (plate 4); any blue light emanating from the subject is brought to a focus 0.5 mm in front of the retina and therefore forms a blurry blue image on it. One way to take advantage of chromatic aberration is for the eye to place photoreceptors sensitive to light of different colors at different distances from the lens, a solution adopted by certain fish (Land & Nilsson 2002).

Using modern equipment, the *optical imperfections* in the structure of the cornea and lens can be measured precisely using *adaptive optics* (Roorda

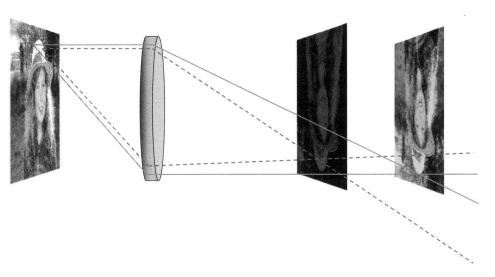

Figure 2.8 (plate 4)
Chromatic aberration. Light reflected from a single point contains a mixture of colors, represented here simply as yellow and blue. Light of different colors gets bent to a different extent, with blue being bent more than yellow. Consequently, if the lens focuses yellow from the subject onto the retina then blue light from the subject forms a perfectly focused image 0.5 mm in front of the retina. This blue light therefore forms a fuzzy image by the time it reaches the retina.

2011). Once these imperfections are known, it is possible to work out what the image on the retina looks like. This has been done for the letter "E" in figure 2.9, and it is clear that the retinal image is far from perfect. However, there is evidence that each eye can compensate for its own particular optical imperfections (Roorda 2011). Even so, given that the image shown in figure 2.9 is the image formed by a normal eye, it seems remarkable that we see as well as we do.

The photoreceptors in the mammalian retina point toward the *back* of the eye, so that the nerve fiber attached to each photoreceptor has to run along the *surface* of the retina. Consequently, the light rays that contribute to the retinal image have to pass through this layer of nerve fibers before reaching the light-sensitive photoreceptors. These rays also have to pass through blood vessels that run across the surface of the retina, as shown in figure 2.10. However, blood vessels skirt around the most sensitive part of the retina, the central fovea. The back-to-front retinal design also ensures that the nerve fibers converge in a bundle at a single point before passing through the retina to reach the brain. This is the cause of the classic *blind*

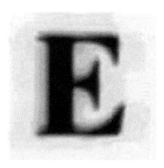

Figure 2.9
Image of the letter "E" as it would appear on the retina is distorted, due to optical imperfections in the structure of the cornea and lens. Courtesy David Williams, University of Rochester.

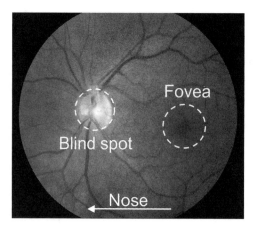

Figure 2.10
Retina, as seen through an ophthalmoscope. The branching structures are arteries and veins lying close to the surface of the retina, which converge on the blind spot (optic disk). The dark region to the right is the fovea, and the nose is to the left of this image. The centers of the blind spot and fovea are 4.3 mm apart. Courtesy Robin Farr.

spot or *optic disk*, shown in figures 2.10 and 2.11. In contrast, an octopus has it photoreceptors the "right way around," which means its nerve fibers form a bundle behind the retina, and so the octopus does not have a blind spot.

Not Blinded by the Light
In bright sunlight, the muscles of the iris contract, and the pupil's diameter is reduced from its maximum diameter of 8 millimeters to 2 millimeters.

(a) (b)

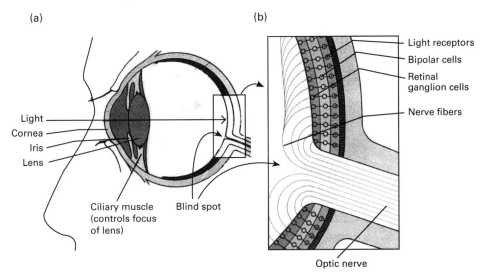

Light receptors
Bipolar cells
Retinal ganglion cells

Nerve fibers

Light
Cornea
Iris
Lens

Ciliary muscle (controls focus of lens) Blind spot

Optic nerve

Figure 2.11
Schematic diagram of eye and retina. (a) Vertical cross section of eye, showing the blind spot where the optic nerve exits the eye on the nasal (nose or inner) side of the retina. (b) Expansion of inset in (a) to show the three main layers of cells: receptors, bipolars, and ganglion cells. From Frisby & Stone 2010.

This implies that the total area of the pupil shrinks from 50 square millimeters to 3 square millimeters (recall that the area A of a circle with radius r is given by $A = \pi r^2$, where r is half the diameter). This reduction in size amounts to a factor of about 17 (50 ÷ 3), so the eye admits about 17 times more light when the pupil is fully open (e.g., in a dimly lit room) than it does when it's open the least, as in sunlight. But the eye operates over an enormous range of lighting conditions, from moonlight to sunlight, a range that can vary by a factor of 10^{10} (10 billion). Such a range cannot possibly be accommodated by changing the pupil area by a factor of 17. So this simple bit of mathematics suggests that the pupil contributes *relatively* little to the eye's ability to compensate for changes in lighting conditions.

So, why, you might ask, does the pupil get smaller in sunlight? It probably involves the dilemma faced by the *Nautilus*, that is, how to keep the retinal image as sharply focused, yet also as bright, as possible. Indeed, as any amateur photographer knows, a small pupil (aperture) size ensures that objects remain in focus over a wide range of depths from the camera. This is because, as the aperture shrinks, the camera functions increasingly like a pinhole camera. And, just as the image in a pinhole camera is always in focus, so a small pupil ensures that the retinal image is as sharp as possible. In addition, even though the lens of the eye does a reasonable job of focusing the image on the retina, as we have seen in figure 2.9, optical imperfections in the structure of the cornea and lens introduce distortions, which are reduced as the pupil shrinks. So the eye tries to set the pupil size to be small enough to keep the retinal image in focus and relatively unaffected by lens imperfections, but also large enough to ensure the image is bright. Although this trade-off between sharpness and brightness can result in an image that is both bright and sharp, under a moonlit sky, the pupil will open up, yielding a retinal image that's neither sharp nor bright.

These conclusions are based on observations about pupil size and light levels and on simple mathematical calculations. In subsequent chapters, we will often see how a combination of observation and mathematics can be used to obtain insights into why the visual system operates as it does.

The Retina
In a typical human eye, the image is brought to a focus 16 millimeters behind the lens onto the retina. Unlike the sensor array or film frame of a camera, the retina does not have a uniform covering of photoreceptors. The dark spot to the right in figure 2.10 is the *macula*, which is about 5 mm across and contains a yellow pigment that blocks ultraviolet light. Within the macula, there is a small circular region about 0.5 mm in diameter (1.7 degrees), the *fovea* (Latin for "pit"), packed with color-sensitive photoreceptors called *cones*. Within the fovea, cones are densely packed at about 200,000 per square millimeter, and this is the place where we see in greatest detail.

There are three types of cones, which are sensitive to long (red), medium (green) and short (blue) wavelengths of light, but the fovea contains only cones sensitive to long and medium wavelengths. Indeed, about half of all cones sensitive to red and green wavelengths within the retina are packed into the foveal area, and the overall proportions of cones sensitive to red, green, and blue light are 63, 31, and 6 percent, respectively (although recent evidence suggests these figures vary between individuals). Whereas the blue cone pigment originates from a phylogenetically primordial subsystem, the red and green cone pigments evolved more recently from a common ancestor, about 35 million years ago.

Outside the fovea, the proportion of cones decreases and the proportion of another receptor type, the *rods*, increases, as shown in figure 2.12. Whereas cones are relatively insensitive, rods are exquisitely sensitive and

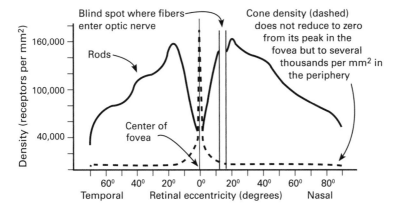

Figure 2.12

Rod and cone densities across the retina of the left eye. Approximate distribution of cones and rods showing how their densities vary with retinal eccentricity. The nasal and temporal sides of the retina are on the same side as the nose and temple, respectively. From Frisby & Stone 2010.

operate only in low-light conditions. In fact, rods are essentially "bleached out" by normal daylight and do not contribute to vision under such conditions.

Rods and cones rely on the presence of different forms of a photosensitive pigment, *opsin*, in order to detect light. Remarkably, all eyes in the animal kingdom rely on different forms of the same basic *opsin* pigment. This suggests that, even though eyes have evolved many times in many different species, they all derive their photosensitive pigments from a single primordial genetic source.

In the dark, the outside of a photoreceptor is 35 millivolts (mV) more positive than its inside, so it is said to have a "negative resting membrane potential" of –35mV. In contrast, the photoreceptors of invertebrates (e.g., spiders, squid, and snails) have a *positive* resting potential, which suggests that it is the flow of information, not electrons, that matters.

Light striking the millions of light-sensitive molecules within a (vertebrate) photoreceptor changes the configuration of its opsin pigments. These changes are analogous to those imposed on light-sensitive films of old (non-digital) cameras, and the image of a scene is recorded by the retina much as it is on those films. Using the eye as a kind of biological camera, in 1878, Wilhelm Kühne took advantage of this to reveal the exact nature of the image projected onto the retina of a rabbit after it had been looking at a scene for some time, as shown in figure 2.13.

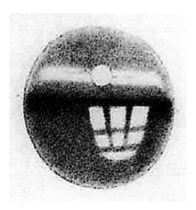

Figure 2.13
Optogram. The last thing ever seen by a rabbit is the image imprinted on its retina by the scene in front of it. Recorded by Wilhelm Kühne in 1878.

The cascade of chemical processes that follows from light being absorbed by a photoreceptor results in its membrane voltage becoming even more negative, a process known as "hyperpolarization." For reasons we will not explore, this decreases the flow of chemical neurotransmitters that normally inhibit the activity of the cells receiving inputs from photoreceptors. The most important of these cells are the *retinal ganglion cells*.

Unlike photoreceptors, retinal ganglion cells do not simply mirror the inputs from photoreceptors, but release volleys of spikes or *action potentials* along their output lines. The difference between the graded voltage outputs of photoreceptors and the spikes of ganglion cells marks a change from the *analog* to the *digital* world. As we'll see in chapter 3, Logan's theorem (1977) suggests that this change is vital for efficient transmission of information in any system, including telephones, satellites, and brains.

What the Eye Does not Tell the Brain
A digital camera contains about 10 million photosensitive elements, each of which corresponds to one picture element, or *pixel*, in a digital photograph, as shown in figure 2.14. In contrast, the retina contains 126 million photoreceptors, each of which measures the amount of light at one point in the retinal image. However, the *optic nerve*, which exits via the back of the eye on its way to the brain, contains only one million fibers (see figure 2.11). At first, this seems to imply that the eye is not telling the brain everything it knows because it looks as if less than 1 percent (1/126) of the

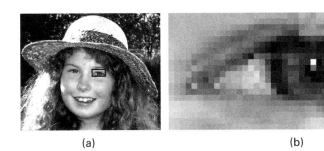

(a)   (b)

Figure 2.14
Pixels. (a) Digital image consisting of picture elements or *pixels*. (b) Zooming in on
the boxed area in (a) reveals individual pixels. Each pixel has a specific gray level,
which is the output of a single photoreceptor and can be represented as a number
(typically between 0 and 255). Similarly, each photoreceptor (rod or cone) in the
retina has an output that corresponds to the amount of light within the corresponding small patch of the retinal image.

information in the retinal image gets sent to the brain. However, as we
will discover, what the eye does not tell the brain, the brain does not need
to know.

A clue as to why the eye does not tell the brain everything can be found
inside any digital camera. Even though a typical digital image consists of
10 million pixels, most images take up only about 2 million pixels worth
of space when stored inside the camera or on a computer. What happens
to the other 8 million pixels' worth of data?

A class of techniques known as "image compression" effectively squeezes
out all unnecessary data from the image, leaving a compressed version that
can contain all of the information in the original image. Provided the
method used to compress the original image is known, it can easily be
reconstituted in its full, 10-million-pixel glory. This is precisely what
happens when the stored version of an image is viewed as 10 million pixels
on a computer monitor.

The fact that a typical image can be compressed by a factor of 5 suggests
that most of the information in the image is *redundant*. For example, the
information in almost any single pixel is similar to that in neighboring
pixels, so most of the information in a single pixel is implicit in the pixels
around it. The similarity between neighboring pixels occurs because, for
example, the sky is about the same shade of blue almost everywhere across
an image, and skin tones change only very slowly across an image. For
some images, almost all of the pixels are the same color, as in figure 2.15.

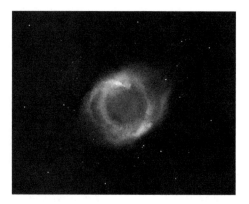

Figure 2.15
Helix nebula, which resembles an eye floating in space, is a gaseous envelope expelled by a dying star. Photographs taken by the Hubble telescope are compressed before being transmitted to Earth and then decompressed to recover their original images. Courtesy NASA.

So if the color of one pixel is known, it's pretty likely that its neighbors have similar colors, not always, but most of the time.

The precise mechanism by which the eye removes redundant information from the retinal image will be explored in chapter 3. For now, it is sufficient to appreciate that the eye does not tell the brain the light intensity at every point in the retinal image because the structure of natural images is massively redundant; the brain does not need to know such details. It is this redundancy that allows very large images to be transmitted in compressed form from a camera to a computer, from Australia to the United States, from the Hubble telescope to Earth, and from the eye to the brain.

3   The Neuronal Machinery of Vision

The distortions introduced by the retina seem to be meaningful; the retina is acting
as a filter rejecting unwanted information and passing useful information.
—Horace Barlow (1953)

Impressions

*Vast plains of gray, a virtual famine of information, a desert bereft even of
redundant data. An arc of pure light sears itself into the retina, abutting an arc
of darkness, creating a long cliff edge of light, and the famine is over. The edge
is swallowed whole by the swarms of light-hungry photoreceptors, and finally
digested by retinal neurons waiting to gorge on their daily fill of light-candy data.
They spew the Logan-remnants of that mere data at the patient brain in the form
of pure information. In its own time, assured by its own computational competence, the brain builds a world from the sparse spikes spat from the eye, bit by
bit, byte by byte, until there is no doubt that the retina betrayed its image when
it stole that light from the world.*

Neurons and Wineglasses

A neuron is like a wineglass. Just as a wineglass "sings along" or *resonates*
with a specific musical note, so a neuron "resonates" by increasing its firing
rate in response to specific patterns of light that change over both space
and time on the retina. In its simplest form, such a pattern can be a spot
of light, a moving spot, or a series of moving stripes. At its most complex,
a pattern can consist of a photograph of, say, Jennifer Aniston (in the TV
series *Friends*; see "Inferotemporal Cortex" in chapter 4). And just as a
wineglass can resonate to a specific note even in the midst of a cacophony
of other notes, so a neuron can detect the presence of its preferred pattern
in the midst of a complex retinal image.

In fact, every physical object has its own resonant pattern, which usually takes the form of a specific note or frequency. As with a wineglass, this resonant frequency can be discovered by simply tapping the object. For example, if you tap a bookcase with your fingernail then the sound you hear is different from the one you hear when you tap a desk or table. This is because tapping an object forces it to respond with its own particular resonant frequency. But the resonant frequency of an object is a *fixed* property of that object. (Most objects have a small range of similar preferred frequencies, with the object's resonant frequency at the center of this range—just as most neurons respond to a small range of patterns that are similar to their preferred ones).

In contrast, the special trick that the brain has pulled off is the ability to *learn*, so that the pattern of light, color, and motion to which a neuron responds can change with experience. This ensures that every part of a retinal image is confronted with a battery of neurons, each tuned to a specific pattern. The resultant set of neuronal activations effectively translates the retinal image from the language of light intensities to the language of neuronal firings.

On the one hand, the general accuracy of this translation is remarkable, inasmuch as there is very little loss of information between the retinal image and the neuronal representation of that image (Rieke et al. 1997; Nemenman et al. 2008). On the other hand, when the translation fails, the particular way it fails gives rise to the many visual illusions we experience, most of which are predictable, and some of which are even desirable (e.g., figure 1.10), when considered in the context of perception.

Neurons

As we have already seen, the brain's fundamental information processing structure is the *neuron*, first described in the beautiful drawings of Santiago Ramón y Cajal in 1910 (figure 3.1). A neuron is a specialized, elongated cell, which acts a little like an electrical cable. It receives inputs through a bushy structure consisting of many filament-like structures or *dendrites*, which together make up the *dendritic tree* and converge on the *cell body*. The neuron's output is delivered through a long, cable-like structure called an "axon," typically 1 micrometer in diameter (a human hair is about 80 micrometers in diameter). Axons in the human body can be a meter or more long, like the ones that connect the base of the spine to the foot.

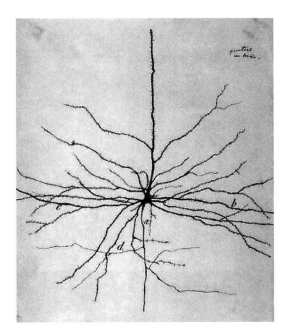

Figure 3.1
Neuron. Ramón y Cajal's drawing from 1910.

A neuron is an elongated bag of salty fluid, enclosed in a membrane punctuated with tiny hatches or *ion channels*. The membrane maintains a voltage difference between the inside and outside of the neuron. Because the outside of the neuron is at a higher voltage than the inside by 70 millivolts (mV), this *resting potential* is by convention given a minus sign (–70 mV). The ion channels in the membrane can open and close according to the voltage across the membrane, and these are essential for the propagation of action potentials, described below.

The first and simplest neuron evolved around 580 million years ago, and its direct descendants can be found coordinating the rhythmic swimming of jellyfish. The neuron represents a step change in communication speed; before its evolution, information was transmitted within organisms by the diffusion of chemical messengers. It's probably no coincidence that most such organisms were slime molds and simple sponges, whose small bodies lack a nervous system. To feed and maintain a large body, good communication between different parts of the body is essential.

Action Potentials, Telephone Cables, and Information Spikes

While the fundamental structural unit of the brain is the neuron, the currency of the brain is the *action potential* or *spike*, which travels at *conduction velocities* from 1 to 120 meters (3 to 380 feet) per second (figure 3.2). If we take a single neuron and gradually increase its input (by injecting a small current into it) then at first no output appears on its axon. If you increase the input still further, a threshold is breached (at around –55 mV), which results in a rapid and transient decrease in the voltage across its membrane. This localized spike of decreased voltage opens a self-propagating bow wave of voltage changes—the *action potential*—that travels along the neuron's axon and has a height of 0.1 volt in amplitude, as shown in figure 3.2.

Edgar Adrian (1926) was the first to discover that, if the input to a neuron is increased by applying pressure to the skin, for example then the number of action potentials per second or *firing rate* increases with the pressure. This is true of *all* neurons: an increase in stimulation, whether through touch, sight (e.g., contrast), or hearing, produces an increase in

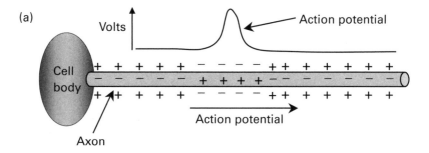

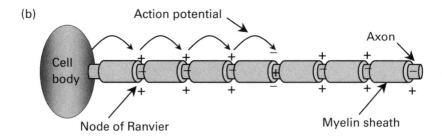

Figure 3.2
Action potential. (a) Axon of a neuron actively propagates a localized change in voltage (action potential) along its length. (b) If an insulating myelin sheath is wrapped around the axon then the action potential propagates by "jumping" between gaps in the myelin sheath.

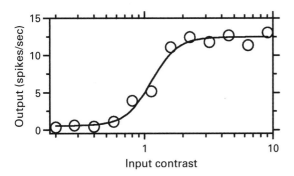

Figure 3.3
Nonlinear encoding. As the amount of input to a neuron increases, its output firing rate increases in a typical S-shaped or sigmoidal curve. Circles represent data points, which have been fitted with the curve shown, which is the neuron's input/output or *transfer function*. The neuron was from marmoset visual cortex, and the input was measured in terms of luminance contrast. Reproduced with permission from Persi et al. 2011.

the firing rate of neurons in the corresponding sensory system as shown in figure 3.3.

Exponential Decay

An action potential requires energy to maintain its journey along the neuron's axon. This is because any passive wave, such as a wave on water or an electrical signal in a cable, dissipates its energy as it travels, becoming progressively weaker with distance from its origin. If the distance between the origin and the final destination is short then this weakening effect is relatively small. But if the distance is large then the signal may be lost almost entirely, as it gradually becomes indistinguishable from the random fluctuations present in any medium.

Because each centimeter of axon is no different from any other, the *proportion* of signal lost in the first centimeter is the same as the proportion lost in the second. Imagine, for example, that a spike consisting of a short pulse of electricity with an amplitude (height) of 100 mV loses half its energy for every centimeter of axon traveled. Thus, at the end of the first centimeter, the pulse has an amplitude of 50 mV (1/2 × 100 mV), and at end the second centimeter, an amplitude of 25 mV (1/2 × 50 mV). By the end of the third centimeter, the amplitude is again halved, yielding a wave with an amplitude of 12.5 mV (1/2 × 25 mV), and so on.

The loss of a constant proportion of amplitude for every centimeter traveled results in an *exponential decay* in signal amplitude. After traveling 100 centimeters, the signal has an amplitude of very nearly zero (about 10^{-30} or 0.000000000000000000000000000001 mV). The point is that any signal that decays at an exponential rate has an amplitude not much greater than zero after long distances, even if the rate of exponential decay is relatively modest. For example, if we replace the 50 percent fall in amplitude along each centimeter with a fall of 10 percent, then a journey of 100 centimeters would reduce an initial amplitude of 100 mV to 0.003 mV. This is exactly the problem that confronted engineers attempting to lay undersea telephone cables across the Atlantic Ocean; and much of the mathematics that describes how electricity flows through such cables also applies to the flow of electrical currents along axons.

Signal Boosters
The first models of passive propagation of electrical signals through an axon were based on engineering solutions to the problem of transatlantic communication. As is often the case, the solution devised by engineers was similar to the one devised by evolution through natural selection: they placed signal boosters or repeaters at regular intervals along the cable, in order to boost the amplitude of signals enough to be detected and boosted by the next repeater. Using the same principle, evolution foreshadowed this in two ways: first, by effectively having a repeater at *every* point along the axon; second, by having a repeater at regular intervals along the axon. Initiating a spike sets in train a positive feedback effect that keeps the spike traveling along the neuron's axon with no loss in amplitude overall. A typical neuron maintains a fixed *resting voltage* across its membrane of −70 mV, essentially by ensuring there are more positively charged ions outside than inside (an *ion* is an atom that carries a charge because it has either too many or too few electrons). A spike involves a local increase in voltage across the neuron membrane, and this voltage change opens up voltage-sensitive ion channels that pepper the membrane and act as temporary "hatches." Once open, these ion channels allow sodium ions to flood into the neuron, causing the voltage across the neuron membrane to increase further, and this, in turn, opens ion channels farther along the neuron. As the voltage changes from −70 mV, passes through zero, and then approaches +40 mV, another set of ion channels allows potassium ions to flood out of the neuron, which effectively resets the membrane to its resting voltage of −70 mV. The end result of this positive feedback is a wave in the form of a single spike that travels along the neuron.

The process just described is called "action potential conduction" and refers to neurons that do *not* have a *myelin sheath*. Such neurons are like underground electrical cables that, lacking insulation, allow some current to leak away into the surrounding earth. In contrast, neurons that do have a myelin sheath are effectively insulated against such leakage. However, just as a signal will eventually fade even in an insulated cable, so neurons have repeaters placed at regular intervals, each of which corresponds to a small gap in the insulating sheath. Each section of myelin sheath consists of a *Schwann cell*, which wraps itself around the neuron's axon. Between consecutive Schwann cells, there's a small gap called a "node of Ranvier." Because the axon is insulated everywhere except at the nodes, ions can flood in and out only at the nodes. Once an action potential is set in motion at a single node, passive conduction to the next node ensures the appearance of an action potential at the next node. The action potential thus appears to jump from node to node, a form of conduction called "saltatory conduction" (from Latin *saltare* for "jump" or "dance"). Of course, if a section of myelinated axon were too long then the voltage change at the next node would be insufficient to cause an action potential there, and evolution seems to have erred on the side of caution by making these sections shorter than strictly necessary (typically, 1–2 millimeters long).

The myelin sheath confers two key advantages on a neuron. First, action potentials in myelinated neurons are fast (these are the ones that travel at 120 meters per second or 270 miles per hour). Second, because the ion flows that accompany an action potential occur only at the gaps between insulated sections—at the nodes of Ranvier—once the action potential has passed, the energy to put all those ions back on the right side of the neuron membrane need be applied only there. In contrast, a neuron lacking a myelin sheath needs to move ions back across its membrane at *every* point along the membrane once the action potential has passed.

Before we leave the topic of axons, we should note that, in terms of Marr's framework (introduced in chapter 1), the brain and telephone engineers confronted the same computational problem, and they both found the same computational solution (signal boosters). Whereas the engineers implemented their signal boosters using electronic amplifiers, the brain implements its boosters using a metabolically active cable that can regenerate action potentials at the nodes of Ranvier. This is a neat example of how different systems, when confronted with the same computational problem, can benefit from the same type of solution, even as they make use of different machinery (implementations) in each case.

Synapses

Neurons communicate with one another across small gaps called "synapses" (figure 3.4). Information is conveyed in the form of action potentials from many (sometimes thousands) of *presynaptic* neurons. Converging on a single *postsynaptic* neuron, these action potentials release chemical *neurotransmitters*, which diffuse across the synapse and, in binding to special *receptors* on the postsynaptic neuron, alter its membrane voltage. If enough neurotransmitter is released then a voltage *threshold* in the postsynaptic neuron is breached, and the positive feedback described above ensures that an action potential is initiated in the postsynaptic neuron. This neuron, in turn, then contributes to the firing of action potentials in

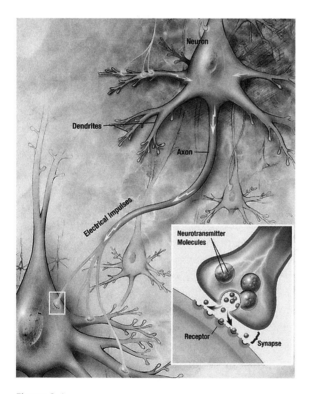

Figure 3.4
Synapse. Each neuron receives inputs via its dendrites. If these inputs are sufficiently large then an output in the form of an action potential appears in the neuron's axon. This causes chemical neurotransmitter to be released at the synapses to other neurons. Courtesy Creative Commons.

other neurons. Thus a single image on the retina gives rise to graded photoreceptor outputs that are converted to action potentials, which yield a
cascade of activated neurons within the brain. At a neuronal level of explanation, that's how the brain sees the world.

The Cost of Neuronal Computation

Neurons are expensive devices in terms of their overall energy demands.
About 13 percent of the brain's supply of energy is used for sending signals
down neurons, and the rest is for maintenance. The energy costs of a single
spike are such that this 13 percent can support an average firing rate of
only 0.16 spikes/second for each neuron in the neocortex (and the neocortex uses about 44 percent of the brain's overall energy). More importantly, this type of analysis suggests that the luxury of having a big brain
incurs two related energy costs. First, there is the substantial cost of main-
taining neurons in their resting state. Second, there is the cost of actually
using one of these expensive devices, a cost that is so high that we can
afford to use only 2–4 percent of them at any one time (Lennie 2003).

Horseshoe Crabs, Computation, Frogs, and Cats

Having inserted a microelectrode into a neuron in a frog's retina, Horace
Barlow (1953), a pioneer in visual neuroscience, shone a light into the
frog's eye. The neuron, which had, up until that moment, been producing
spikes at a steady rate of 20 per second, increased its rate momentarily, and
then resumed firing at 20 spikes per second. Barlow would have been less
than surprised if he had observed such a relatively unexciting result in the
foregoing imaginary scenario. Barlow went on to describe how ganglion
cells in the frog retina seem to respond to "interesting" spots of light (e.g.,
ones that move), and, in the same year, Stephen Kuffler (1953) made a
similar discovery in the visual system of the cat.

The fact that two very different species, the frog and the cat, seemed to
demonstrate similar visual responses to spots of light, though intriguing,
could be attributed to chance. As early as 1949, H. Keffer Hartline, had
shown that photoreceptors in the eye of the horseshoe crab *Limulus*
responded best, not to the total amount of light, but to local *changes*
in light intensity (e.g., to spots of light). Taken together, these discoveries
by Hartline, Barlow, and Kuffler involved not just three species, but three
different animal classes (four taxonomic levels *above* species): Meros-
tomata (a class of arthropods), Amphibia (amphibians), and Mammalia
(mammals).

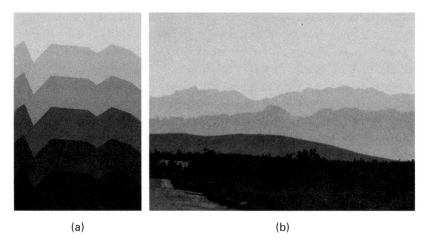

(a)   (b)

Figure 3.5
Naturalistic portrayal of the Chevreul illusion (see figure 3.6a). The light region just
above each hilltop and the dark region just below each hilltop are illusory. (a) Syn-
thetic image with same luminance profile as in figure 3.6a demonstrates illusion.
(b) Photograph of hills. Image courtesy of Alan Stubbs.

Horace Barlow has described vision as the detection of suspicious coin-
cidences. If the same criterion applies to the search for general principles
of vision then the cross-species coincidence described above is certainly
suspicious. Indeed, the horseshoe crab, the frog, and the cat all possess
cells that respond in a similar manner to changes in luminance; so much
so that all three species almost certainly experience the *Chevreul illusion*,
shown in figures 3.5 and 3.6.

In figure 3.5a, each jagged horizontal stripe has a single *uniform* gray
level. This can be seen more clearly in figure 3.6a, where the steplike profile
has been overlaid on the corresponding vertical stripes. In both cases, an
illusory dark narrow region is seen just before the transition from a dark to
a light stripe, and an *illusory* light narrow region is seen just after each
dark-to-light transition, as indicated by the curve overlaid on figure 3.6b.

We'll explore below how these different species, which make use of different visual machinery, manage to see the same illusion. For now, notice
that the visual task is pretty much identical in each case. In terms of David
Marr's computational framework, all three species have found different
materials and (as we will see) different methods to achieve the same end
result. Let's begin by considering how Hartline's discoveries about the
horseshoe crab suggest that it sees the Chevreul illusion.

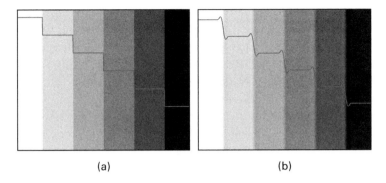

(a)   (b)

Figure 3.6

(a) Chevreul illusion, where luminance profile is shown by the solid line as a series of steps. (b) Chevreul illusion in (a) as seen through the eye of the horseshoe crab, with the solid line showing the small luminance dips and bumps perceived at each step edge.

The Illusory Vision of the Horseshoe Crab

The horseshoe crab *Limulus* has a compound eye, similar in design to that of most insects and modern crabs. The eye consists of many *ommatidia*, tube-like photoreceptors, each of which acts like a short length of optic fiber, channeling light down to a few light-sensitive cells at the base of the ommatidium. The tubelike structure of an ommatidium ensures that it's sensitive only to light from a small range of directions, and this, in turn, ensures that the entire array of ommatidia has outputs which form a rough picture of the scene before it.

H. Keffer Hartline and Clarence Graham (1932) discovered how to record from single nerve fibers emanating from the eye of *Limulus*, and this, in itself, was no mean feat. But, as is often the case, the seeds of Hartline's key discoveries in 1949 were hidden in small, unexplained side effects of the experimental setup. "When I first worked with Limulus," Hartline (1967) noted in his Nobel lecture (p274), "I thought that the receptor units [ommatidia] acted independently of one another. But I soon noticed that extraneous lights in the laboratory, rather than increasing the rate of discharge of impulses from a receptor, often caused a decrease in its activity. Neighboring ommatidia, viewing the extraneous room lights more directly than the receptor on which I was working, could inhibit that receptor quite markedly."

As a result of those early informal observations, Hartline discovered that the output of a single photoreceptor *decreased* if a spot of light was shone on any nearby photoreceptor. Thus it seemed as if the array of photoreceptors in the horseshoe crab eye, rather than simply mirroring the structure of the scene before it, distorted the "image" that was sent to the horseshoe crab's brain through some sort of interactions between the individual photoreceptors. In 1958, Hartline and Floyd Ratliff would publish a mathematical model of those interactions.

Hartline found that each photoreceptor has connections from nearby photoreceptors, and that, if these connections were cut then the response of each photoreceptor depended *only* on the amount of light entering that photoreceptor, and not on the light entering neighboring photoreceptors. In essence, Hartline discovered that each photoreceptor had mutually inhibitory connections with its neighbors. Specifically, he found that the amount of inhibition exerted by photoreceptor A on another photorecep-tor B depended on the distance between them, and Robert Barlow (1967) discovered that this inhibition peaked at a distance of two to four omma-tidia. The net effect of this mutual inhibition between photoreceptors is to exaggerate differences in luminance, so that a *step edge* in luminance gets transformed into a wave with a peak and trough on either side of the step edge, as shown in figure 3.7.

The reason for this wave-like response can be understood by examining the outputs of pairs of photoreceptors at different points along a step edge. In figure 3.8a, both photoreceptors A and B are exposed to the lighter part of the step edge, so both have a high input. However, both A and B inhibit each other in proportion to the amount of input each of them receives, the net effect of this high input and high mutual inhibition is a low output from both A and B.

In figure 3.8b, the photoreceptors C and D straddle the luminance edge. The photoreceptor C is exposed to the lighter part of the step edge and so has a high input, whereas photoreceptor D is exposed to the darker part of the step edge and so has a low input. The upshot is that the massive inhibitory effect from C depresses D's output to a level well below what it would be otherwise, which explains why D has a very low output.

But why does C have such a large output? Consider the photoreceptor A, buried in the middle of the bright strip. Just like C, the photoreceptor A has a high input, but, unlike C, the brightly lit photoreceptor A receives massive inhibition from *all* of its brightly lit neighbors. In contrast, C receives much less inhibition, because half of its neighbors lie in the darker strip and therefore provide very little inhibition to C. Thus the high input to C and a relative lack of inhibition from half of its (poorly lit) neighbors conspire to boost the output of C.

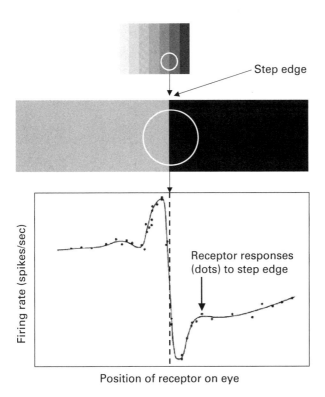

Step edge

Receptor responses
(dots) to step edge

Firing rate (spikes/sec)

Position of receptor on eye

Figure 3.7
(Top) Chevreul illusion. (Middle) Close-up of one edge. (Bottom) Solid curve was
fitted through the measured outputs (dots) of photoreceptors at different positions
across the edge. Reproduced with permission from Barlow 1967.

In figure 3.8c, both photoreceptors E and F are exposed to the darker
part of the step edge, so both have a low input. Although, as with other
neighboring photoreceptors, both E and F inhibit each other in proportion
to the amount of input each of them receives, because their inputs
are small, their inhibitory effect on each other is also small. The net effect
of this low input and low mutual inhibition is a low output from both
E and F. Thus the net overall effect of this mutual inhibition by photoreceptors on either side of a step edge is to exaggerate the magnitude of
that edge. (The data shown in figure 3.7 is from the horseshoe crab eye,
whereas the data in figure 3.8 is idealized based on the assumption that
uniform illumination at any level yields the same low output from
photoreceptors.)

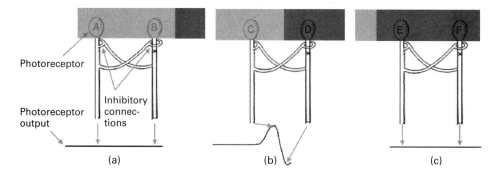

Figure 3.8

(a–c) Responses of pairs of photoreceptors at different positions on a step edge of the Chevreul illusion. Photoreceptors within each pair are assumed to be separated by two to four photoreceptors, a distance at which there is a maximum inhibitory effect of each photoreceptor on its neighbors. Thus the graph in (b) depicts the outputs of several photoreceptors between the peak and trough shown. Together, these define the overall responses shown in figure 3.7.

The horseshoe crab's visual system is one of the few systems for which a precise mathematical model exists, which accounts for the measured outputs in the figures above. Hartline's Nobel Prize was at least partly a result of choosing a system simple enough to be investigated with relatively crude techniques, but complex enough to exemplify the general principles by which any visual system detects salient features in the visual world.

Receptive Fields and Mexican Hats

For a neuron to respond to light in a particular part of the retinal image, it seems self-evident that the neuron must be connected, either directly or through other neurons, to photoreceptors in that part of the image. Residing inside the retina are neurons called "retinal ganglion cells" (see figure 2.11), each of which has its own small population of photoreceptors, so that its output is affected by light that falls within a small, roughly circular region on the retina—the *receptive field*. Outside of this region, light has little or no effect on the ganglion cell's output.

The particular way that a spot of light affects a given ganglion cell not only defines the overall shape of a receptive field; it also defines the internal *structure* of that receptive field, as shown in figure 3.9. Both Horace Barlow (1953) and Stephen Kuffler (1953) found that a spot of light in the

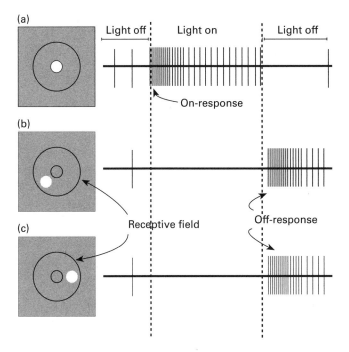

Figure 3.9

Receptive field. Schematic diagram of responses of a ganglion cell with an on-center receptive field. (a) Spot of light in the central excitatory region causes an initial burst of action potentials, followed by a high rate of discharge, which ceases when the light is turned off. (b, c) Light anywhere in the annulus inhibits the firing rate, reducing it from a baseline firing rate to about zero spikes per second. A rebound burst of activity is observed when this inhibitory effect is removed as the light is switched off. From Frisby & Stone 2010.

center of a receptive field yielded the highest firing rate from a ganglion cell. As they moved the spot in a straight line away from the center, the firing rate diminished until it reached a resting or *baseline firing rate* (e.g., 5 spikes/second). But as they moved the spot farther away from the center, the firing rate first fell below this baseline level and then returned to it. Moreover, they obtained an almost identical profile no matter in which direction they moved the spot of light. Thus they found that the receptive field structure resembles a Mexican hat (sombrero), as shown in figure 3.10, a type of circular receptive field called "on-center." A complementary "off-center" receptive field has exactly the "opposite" characteristics: its ganglion cell is inhibited by light at the receptive field center, but excited by

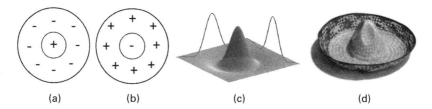

Figure 3.10
Ganglion cell receptive fields. (a) On-center/off-surround. (b) Off-center/on-surround.
(c) Three-dimensional graph showing the sensitivity to light spots placed in different
regions of the receptive field of a cell with an on-center receptive field. The spike
in the middle shows where light excites the cell, and the trough around this spike
shows where light inhibits the cell. (d) These cells are sometimes said to have
Mexican hat receptive fields.

light within the surrounding area known as the "annulus," as shown in
figure 3.10b.

David Hubel (1988, p. 40), a pioneer in modern visual neurophysiology,
put these results in historical perspective: "What is especially interesting
to me is the unexpectedness of the results, as reflected in the failure of
anyone before Kuffler to guess that something like center-surround receptive fields could exist or that the optic nerve would ignore anything so
boring as diffuse light levels." With the benefit of hindsight, and in the
context of findings presented later in this chapter, it seems surprising that
the results were thought to be unexpected. This change in perspective gives
some indication of the progress we've made since those results were first
reported. However, to fully understand the developments that followed,
we first need to know exactly what's meant by *luminance* and *contrast*.

Luminance
Light is measured in *candelas*, a name derived from the fact that, historically, one candle emitted about one candela of light. The *luminance* of a
surface, like a piece of white paper, is the amount of light reflected from
it (figure 3.11), measured in candelas per square meter (cd/m^2). Clearly,
light-colored paper reflects more light than dark-colored paper, so luminance depends on the nature of the surface. Similarly, paper of any color
reflects more light in sunshine than in shade, so luminance also depends
on the ambient light levels.

The amount of light hitting each square meter of a surface, called its
"illuminance," is also measured in candelas per square meter (cd/m^2). The

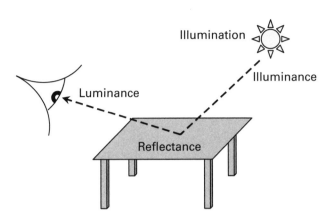

Figure 3.11
Surface *reflectance*. The amount of light reflected per square meter of a surface, its *luminance*, is affected by the ambient *illumination*, and the proportion of light reflected by that surface, its *reflectance* or *albedo*.

proportion of illuminant light reflected by a surface, called its "reflectance" or "albedo," varies from zero to one, and corresponds to the perception of *lightness*. Thus, if a surface is illuminated by 50 cd/m^2 of light and reflects 5 cd/m^2 of light, its reflectance is 5 cd/m^2 ÷ 50 cd/m^2 = 0.1 (10 percent). Finally, just as any bright object appears less bright when viewed at a distance, so the amount of light entering the eye from an object's surface is reduced by the distance (squared) between the surface and the eye.

Contrast
Denoted by the letter C, the *contrast* within a given patch of an image, also called the "Michelson contrast," is the maximum luminance I_{max} minus the minimum luminance I_{min}, all divided by their sum:

$$C = \frac{I_{max} - I_{min}}{I_{max} + I_{min}}.$$

As an example, consider figure 3.12e, where the luminance in the central region is I_{max} and the luminance in the circular surround is I_{min}. If we substitute the luminance values of these regions into the equation above then we find that the images in figure 3.12a and e as well as those in figure 3.12b and d have the same contrast, whereas the image in figure 3.12c has zero contrast.

More important, if we were to present each of the images in these figures to an off-center receptive field then the one in figure 3.12a would yield a

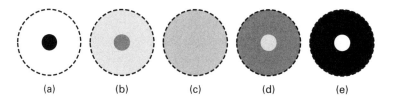

Figure 3.12

Contrast. Images in (a) and (e) have high contrast. The image in (a) would be the preferred stimulus for an off-center ganglion cell, whereas the image in (e) would be the preferred stimulus for an on-center ganglion cell. The image in (b) would increase the firing rate of an off-center cell above its baseline firing rate, while decreasing the firing rate of an on-center cell, and vice versa for the image in (d). The image in (c) has zero contrast, and would elicit no response (i.e., no change in the baseline firing rate) from either type of cell.

high ganglion cell response, whereas the lower-contrast one in figure 3.12b would yield a smaller response. Ideally, the image in figure 3.12c would yield no response, although in practice it would probably give a small transient response, and the images in figure 3.12c and d would both inhibit responses. For an on-center receptive field, exactly the "opposite" set of responses would be obtained, with the highest response evoked by figure 3.12e and the lowest response evoked by figure 3.12a. For convenience, we will use the term *positive contrast* to refer to contrasts such as figure 3.12d and e that excite a ganglion cell with an on-center receptive field and *negative contrast* to refer to contrasts such as figure 3.12a and b that excite a ganglion cell with an off-center receptive field.

Crucially, contrast depends on the *difference* in luminance but is independent of the *amount* of luminance. For example, if the luminance in the center of the receptive field in figure 3.12b is I_{max} = 15 cd/m^2, and the luminance in the surround is I_{min} = 5 cd/m^2 then the contrast is (15 – 5)/20 = 0.5. If the overall luminance increased, perhaps because the sun came out from behind a cloud then both luminance the maximum and minimum levels would increase by the same factor. If the overall luminance increased tenfold then we'd have I_{max} = 150 cd/m^2, and I_{min} = 50 cd/m^2, and so the contrast would remain the *same* at (150 – 50)/200 = 0.5. Thus, if the overall amount of light increases then, even though the luminance *difference* between the center and surround increases, the contrast remains constant. This is not only mathematically convenient; it also mirrors the output of retinal ganglion cells, which usually responds to the luminance contrast between the center and surround of its receptive field, rather than to absolute light levels.

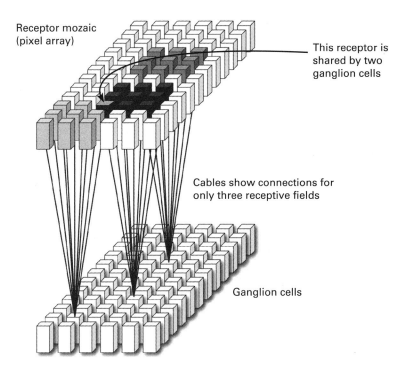

Receptor mozaic
(pixel array)

This receptor is
shared by two
ganglion cells

Cables show connections for
only three receptive fields

Ganglion cells

Figure 3.13
Receptive fields of individual retinal ganglion cells, showing a small amount of overlap. In this example, the overlap results in a single photoreceptor being shared by two receptive fields. From Frisby & Stone 2010.

Tiling the Retina

The receptive fields of ganglion cells effectively tile the retina (Gauthier et al. 2009), and the overlap between adjacent receptive fields means that each photoreceptor can belong to about ten receptive fields, as shown in figure 3.13 (Meister & Berry 1999). As we will see later, there are several types of retinal ganglion cells, and, because each type of ganglion cell tiles the retina, every point on the retina is overlaid with multiple receptive fields (figure 3.14).

The Illusory Vision of the Mexican Hat

Even though there is no direct mutual inhibition between photoreceptors of the vertebrate eye, the structure of an on-center receptive field effectively makes each ganglion cell behave as if it were a photoreceptor in the eye of a horseshoe crab. To understand this, consider the output of

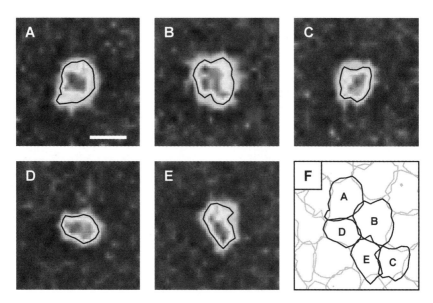

Figure 3.14
Receptive fields of individual on-center (parasol) monkey retinal ganglion cells. The black curves do not indicate the outermost edge of a cell's receptive field, but they do indicate its general shape, so there is overlap between adjacent receptive fields. The white scale bar indicates 0.18 mm on the retina. Other ganglion cell types have receptive fields of different sizes, but each ganglion cell type also tiles the retina. Reproduced with permission from Gauthier et al. 2009.

ganglion cells with receptive fields placed at different points along the luminance edge of two strips within the Chevreul illusion, as shown by the trace in figure 3.15d.

Remember that, because the retina is fully "tiled" with receptive fields, there is an on-center receptive field wherever the luminance edge is on the retina. To simplify this explanation, we will assume that ganglion cells can have *negative* firing rates (this may seem a little odd, but the justification for this simplification is given in a subsequent section).

First, consider a ganglion cell with a receptive field that lies entirely within the light strip, as in figure 3.15a. The excitation caused by the high luminance at the receptive field center is approximately canceled by the inhibition caused by the high luminance in the annulus of the receptive field. Now consider a ganglion cell whose receptive field lies entirely within the dark strip, as in figure 3.15d. The small amount of excitation caused by the low luminance at the receptive field center is effectively canceled by the small amount of inhibition caused by low luminance in the annulus

(a) Receptive field in light yields baseline output.

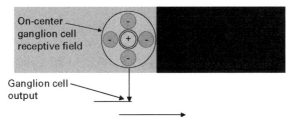

Position of ganglion cell's receptive field on retina

(b) Inhibitory annulus partially in darkness yields high output.

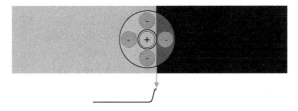

(c) Inhibitory annulus partially in light yields low output.

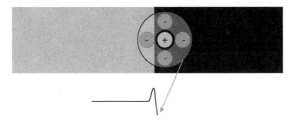

(d) Receptive field in dark region yields baseline output.

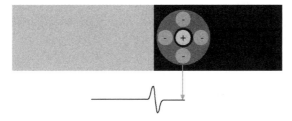

Figure 3.15
Responses of on-center ganglion cells at different positions on a luminance step edge.

of the receptive field. Thus the collective outputs of all ganglion cells with receptive fields that lie entirely within either the dark or light strip define a horizontal line (at baseline firing rate) on either side of the step edge in figure 3.15.

If, however, a ganglion cell's receptive field straddles the light and dark strips then its output changes. Consider a cell that has its excitatory center entirely within the light strip, but part of the inhibitory annulus lies within the dark strip, as shown in figure 3.15b. Because all of the excitatory center is within the light strip, the amount of excitation is high, but because part of the inhibitory annulus receives very little light, it provides very little inhibition on the firing rate of the ganglion cell. The net result of this removal of part of the inhibition is to increase the firing rate of the ganglion cell. Thus the more of the annulus that's in the dark strip, the less inhibition is received by the ganglion cell, and the more its firing rate increases—up to a point. This point is the one depicted in figure 3.15b. A cell with its receptive field slightly to the right of the one shown receives less inhibition, but it also receives less excitation because the excitatory center is now partly in the dark strip. The overall effect of this is to reduce the firing rate of the cell.

If a ganglion cell has its receptive field exactly over the luminance edge (not shown) then the amount of excitation and inhibition balance each other, and the cell's output is at baseline. But because a cell with its receptive field slightly to the right of this perfectly balanced position receives less inhibition from its annulus and even less excitation from its center, its firing rate falls below baseline. For ganglion cells with receptive fields farther to the right, their firing rates continue to fall, reaching a minimum when the excitatory center lies just to the right of the step edge, as in figure 3.15c. At this point, the center receives no light from the lighter strip, and the inhibitory annulus is partly in the light strip, so the ganglion cell receives only inhibition and no excitation. Consequently, the cell's output is very low. For ganglion cells with receptive fields even farther to the right, the amount of inhibition decreases, and the firing rate increases, until finally the entire receptive field is in the dark strip, and the firing rate is once more at baseline, as in figure 3.15d.

Notice that, on average, each square millimeter within the center of the receptive field carries more excitation than the amount of inhibition carried by a square millimeter within the annulus of the receptive field. The reason this must be true is that the relatively large annulus approximately cancels the effects of the smaller center when both are exposed to the same luminance.

The result of this journey across the step edge is a profile of ganglion cell outputs that has roughly the same shape as the firing rates of photo-receptors in the eye of a horseshoe crab (compare figure 3.15 to figure 3.7). At first sight, it looks as if this shape reflects (a) the *difference* in luminance between nearby image points (the contrast), but closer inspection reveals that it represents instead (b) the *difference between the differences* of lumi-nances at nearby pairs of image points (the change in contrast). One consequence is that, for humans and horseshoe crabs, the point where the output curve (the second derivative) passes through the baseline firing rate marks the location of the step edge. Because this baseline corresponds to zero for an equivalent electronic component, the place where the curve passes through baseline is called a "zero-crossing." This will prove impor-tant below.

The fact that the response profiles of photoreceptors in the horse-shoe crab eye and human retinal ganglion cells have the same basic form is remarkable, and not just because it suggests that both humans and horseshoe crabs experience the Chevreul illusion. As was suggested earlier, if species as different as horseshoe crabs, frogs, cats, and humans distort the visual world in the same way then this is probably no coinci-dence. At the very least, these different species manage to generate the same "mistake." But the very different neuronal machinery used by them suggests it's not a mistake caused by the particular hardware within each visual system. In other words, because the visual systems (especially of horseshoe crabs and mammals) are so different from one another, it is probably not a side effect of the physical implementation of the visual system.

This cross-species comparison suggests that the computational task being performed by horseshoe crabs and mammals is the same. If we can find a compelling reason for the existence of the particular characteristics (e.g., experiencing the Chevreul illusion) shared by these visual systems then it seems likely that we would have discovered a general principle of operation for visual systems. More important, because this principle is derived from several species, it transcends the constraints of the particular biological machinery of horseshoe crabs, frogs, and humans. In other words, whatever it is, this principle is unlikely to be a side effect of the quite different physical architecture these species use to build their eyes. Of course, we do not know what this general principle is, but at least we now have some circumstantial evidence that it exists. The nature of this general principle will be explored in the remaining sections of this chapter and in subsequent chapters.

Receptive Field Size and Spatial Scale

The area on the retina of a ganglion cell's receptive field determines whether it responds to luminance changes over a small or large retinal area. For example, if a ganglion cell collates the outputs of, say, 100 photoreceptors that reside within its receptive field with, say, 10 photoreceptors in the central region and 90 in the annulus then it would effectively ignore luminance changes over a very small area (smaller than one or two photoreceptor widths). It would also ignore changes over a large area (larger than 200 photoreceptor widths) because, from the ganglion cell's point of view, a very gradual change in luminance spread over a large area of the retina is pretty much the same as a uniform luminance, and therefore evokes little or no response. Thus ganglion cells have a preferred range of spatial scales, or *spatial frequencies*, over which they can detect changes in luminance.

Spatial Frequency

Spatial frequency is a measure of how "quickly" luminance changes from light to dark from point to point across an image. These changes can be measured either on a surface or in the retinal image. We'll start with a simple example, and then work our way toward the formal definition of spatial frequency.

A pair of black and white stripes, like those on a zebra, represents a change from dark to light. Rather than having stripes with a sudden step change, we can choose to have a gradual change from black to white, as in figure 3.16b. If we were to take a cross section of the luminance in this figure then we would discover a sinuous profile called a "sine wave," as shown in figure 3.17. The distance from the peak of one white stripe to the peak of the next white stripe is called a "cycle" or "period." For example, if the stripes on a zebra were sinusoidal then the wide stripes on its back might yield 2 cycles per millimeter on the page, but the narrow stripes on its face might yield 6 cycles per millimeter.

One way to think of spatial frequency is to imagine yourself driving horizontally across figure 3.16b at a steady speed of, say, 1 centimeter per second. If you were to count the number of luminance peaks whizzing past then you would clearly encounter more peaks if the stripes were narrow than if they were wide. So the *frequency* with which you encounter peaks would increase as the width of stripes was made smaller. In other words, narrow stripes correspond to a *high spatial frequency*, and wide stripes correspond to a *low spatial frequency*.

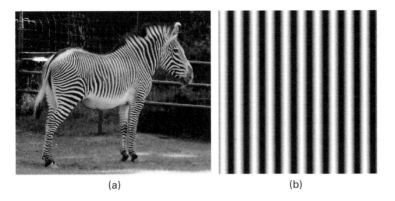

(a)   (b)

Figure 3.16
Spatial frequency. (a) Narrow stripes on the zebra's front leg correspond to a high spatial frequency, whereas wide stripes on its back leg correspond to a low spatial frequency. (b) Grating in which luminance changes gradually in a sinusoidal manner from white to black and back to white. The horizontal distance between contiguous luminance peaks is a single cycle, and the number of cycles per millimeter is a measure of spatial frequency.

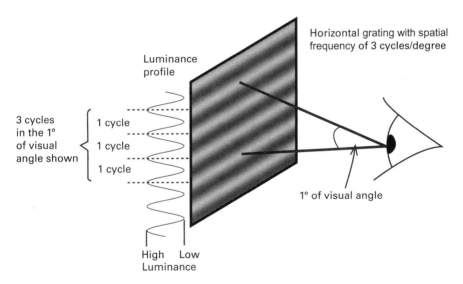

Figure 3.17
Spatial frequency is measured in terms of the number of complete black-white regions (cycles) per degree. From Frisby & Stone 2010.

Of course, because the receptive field exists on the retina rather than on the page, we are really interested in how ganglion cells respond to the size of stripes as measured on the retina. So we should express spatial frequency in terms of cycles per millimeter on the retina, rather than cycles per centimeter on the page. The retinal image of figure 3.16a is much smaller than the photographic image in figure 3.16a. Therefore, in the retinal image, all of the stripes are narrower. For example, the wide stripes on the zebra's back leg might yield 2 cycles per millimeter in the retinal image, but the narrow stripes on its face might yield 6 cycles per millimeter.

Finally, we can translate distance along the retina to a visual angle measured at the lens, so that spatial frequency can be expressed in terms cycles per degree, rather than cycles per millimeter on the retina, as shown in figure 3.17. For comparison, 1 millimeter on the retina corresponds to about 4 degrees of visual angle, and the image of the moon has a diameter of about 1/8 millimeter on the retina and subtends an angle of 0.5 of a degree. The spacing between retinal photoreceptors places a theoretical limit on the highest detectable spatial frequency of about 60 cycles per degree (Roorda 2011).

Fourier Analysis

Considering that he was one of the world's best physicists, Joseph Fourier (1768–1830) was not very good at mathematics. But he had extraordinarily powerful insights into the nature of how the physical world works. This is why he is known as a scientist who could get the right solution to a problem despite getting the details of the mathematics wrong.

As a side effect of working out the distribution of temperature in a heated metal bar, Fourier devised one of the most important techniques in mathematics, which has since become known as "Fourier analysis." In essence, Fourier proved that almost any curve can be decomposed (broken down) into one, and only one, set of sine waves, known as "Fourier components." A *sine wave* is a simple curve that oscillates at a fixed frequency over space or time, as in figure 3.18a–c, and if it is amplified through an audio amplifier then it sounds like a lightly tapped tuning fork. A Fourier analysis of the complicated curve in figure 3.18d would yield the three Fourier components (figure 3.18a–c). In practice, we would need to know the *amplitude* (height) and *phase* (left-right position) of each sine wave component, but this is a detail that need not concern us here. For our purposes, the importance of Fourier analysis is that it can be run either "forward" or "backward." In other words, if a curve can be decomposed

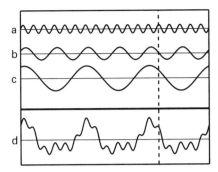

Figure 3.18
Fourier analysis. The complicated curve in (d) is the sum of corresponding points in the sinusoidal curves in (a–c). The height of the dashed line in (d) is the sum of the heights of corresponding points in (a–c). For example, within the dashed line, if the height of the curve in (a) is 0.1, the curve in (b) is 0.01, and the curve in (c) is 0.2, then curve in (d) has a height (0.1 + 0.01 + 0.2) = 0.31 at the dashed line. Conversely, Fourier analysis can be used to decompose the curve in (d) into a unique set of sine waves in (a–c).

into sine waves then it can also be *re*composed by adding those same sine waves back together. In fact, the curve in figure 3.18d was produced by adding together the three sine waves in figure 3.18a–c. For example, the height or *amplitude* of the point in figure 3.18d at the dashed vertical line is the sum of the amplitudes of three corresponding points (also on the dashed line) on the curves in figure 3.18a–c.

Looking at figure 3.18d, you might think that it would be difficult to "unscramble the omelet" and recover the curves in figure 3.18a–c, but that's what Fourier analysis does—it finds the one and only set of sine waves that could have been added together to produce the curve in figure 3.18d. Not every mathematical curve can be produced by adding together just three—or any particular number of—sine waves, but you can always get as close as you like to any curve if you use a sufficiently large number of sine waves.

One method for demonstrating Fourier analysis takes advantage of the idea of resonant frequency introduced at the outset of this chapter. When tapped lightly, a wineglass sounds like a tuning fork because both emit a fairly pure tone, called a "sinusoid." Wineglasses of different sizes emit tones with different frequencies when tapped; these are their *resonant frequencies*. Running a moistened finger around the glass's rim also yields a pure tone, and this has been used since ancient times to play tunes on a

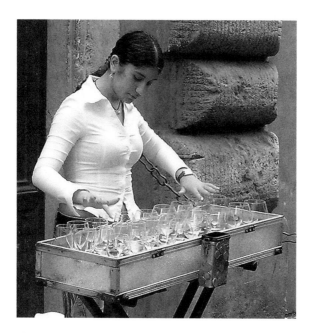

Figure 3.19
Glass harmonica. When a moistened finger is moved around the rim, each glass emits a fairly pure tone, allowing tunes to be played. But when exposed to music, the vibrations set up in each glass allow the glass harmonica to act as a device for performing Fourier analysis. Courtesy Creative Commons.

glass harmonica, as shown in figure 3.19. Conversely, if a wineglass encounters any sound containing its resonant frequency then it vibrates "in sympathy" with that sound, and the amplitude of its vibration is proportional to the amplitude of the sound at the glass's resonant frequency. If that sound is sufficiently loud then the wineglass will shatter.

These sympathetic vibrations mean that a glass harmonica could also be used for Fourier analysis. Suppose a pure tone is played through the speakers of a stereo system in a room containing a glass harmonica. If this tone matches the resonant frequency of a particular glass then that glass, and only that glass, will vibrate. Similarly, if music containing a mixture of many frequencies is played then many (but not all) of the glasses will vibrate, and the amplitude of the vibration for a given glass would be proportional to amplitude of its resonant frequency in the sound coming out of the speakers. Thus each glass effectively "picks out" its own resonant frequency from the complicated sound wave; the amount of vibration of each glass tells us the amplitude of each Fourier component.

In practice, it's difficult to find a wineglass so perfect that it emits a sound that's a pure sine wave, and most glasses emit a mixture of sine waves within a small band of frequencies. This has implications for the sounds that the glass responds to. So, rather than having a single resonant frequency, each glass has a small *bandwidth* of frequencies to which it resonates, and each acts like a temporal *band-pass filter* by ignoring all those frequencies outside this bandwidth.

What, you may ask, has this got to do with vision? Well, just as a sound wave is a complicated curve with an amplitude that varies over *time*, so an image can be considered to be a complicated *surface* that varies over *space*, where this space can be a photograph or the retina, as in figure 3.20b. This is easier to understand if we consider the gray levels in a series of adjacent pixels from an image, as in figure 3.20a. These gray levels define a curve that is not much different from the curve that defines a sound, except that the image gray levels vary in one direction over the space of an image, whereas the sound amplitudes vary over time. But when these two curves are plotted in a graph they are both, from a mathematical perspective, just curves. As such, they are both amenable to Fourier analysis. Thus a Fourier analysis of the curve marked A in figure 3.20a would yield a number of sinusoidal Fourier components with different spatial frequencies. The complexity of this curve suggests that a large number of sinusoidal Fourier

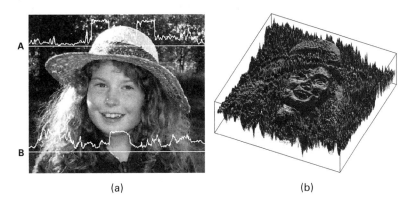

(a)   (b)

Figure 3.20
(a) Image can be represented either by individual pixels in a photograph, where each pixel has a specific gray level, or by photoreceptors in the retina, where each photoreceptor has a specific output voltage (graphs A and B) The gray levels of pixels under each horizontal white line are shown by the graph drawn above it. (b) Image can also be represented as a surface, where the height of each point on the surface is given by the gray level of the corresponding pixel in the image.

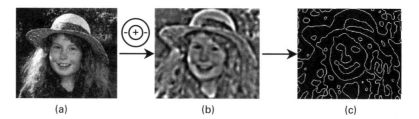

(a)   (b)   (c)

Figure 3.21
(a) Each point in the retinal image is at the center of an on-center retinal ganglion cell. (b) The output of each of these cells is indicated by the gray level at its corresponding location. For example, notice how each eye, which approximates a dark spot against a light background, gives low ganglion cell outputs. (c) Edge map. Each place in (b), where adjacent ganglion cell outputs go from below baseline to above baseline (in any direction across the image) defines a zero-crossing, and corresponds to a luminance edge in (a).

components would be required in this case, but the principle remains the same.

Once we have begun to think of images as consisting of many Fourier components then we can explore how the receptive field of a center-surround ganglion cell essentially "picks out" luminance edges in Fourier components within a particular band of spatial frequencies.

Each point in figure 3.21b shows the output of a model ganglion cell, with high outputs corresponding to light regions and low outputs corresponding to dark regions (the issue of negative cell outputs is addressed in the next section, but, for now, we simply assume that cells can have negative outputs). Crucially, each luminance edge in figure 3.21a forces the ganglion cell outputs to pass through zero, in a manner qualitatively similar to that shown in figure 3.15. Thus each luminance step edge in figure 3.21a is associated with a place in figure 3.21b where the ganglion cell outputs go from below baseline to above baseline (or vice versa); as a reminder, such points are known as "zero-crossings." Each zero-crossing in figure 3.21b has been marked explicitly in the *edge map* shown in figure 3.21c. Thus, in principle, the brain can use the output of ganglion cells to identify the locations of zero-crossings that are the locations of edges in the retinal image.

Notice that each edge found by the ganglion cell's receptive field usually belongs to luminance changes in figure 3.21a over a particular *spatial scale*; things like the hat band. These edges are therefore associated with low spatial frequencies in figure 3.21a. If you now skip ahead to figure 3.25

then the results of processing the image with receptive fields of two different sizes can be seen. The two different edge maps in figure 3.25c are the result of processing the image with receptive fields of two different sizes, each of which acts like a *spatial* band-pass filter. That is, the small receptive field associated with figure 3.25b (left) ignores luminance changes that are spread out over a large image region. Conversely, the large receptive field associated with figure 3.25b (right) ignores each luminance change that is compressed into a small image region. The net result is that each ganglion cell responds best to luminance changes within a reasonably narrow range of spatial frequencies, a range that depends on the size of its receptive field.

Thus, just as each glass in the glass harmonica detects sounds within a specific range of temporal frequencies, so each ganglion cell's receptive field in the retina detects luminance changes over a specific range of spatial frequencies. And, just as the glass harmonica can be viewed as a bank of temporal band-pass filters that essentially performs Fourier analysis on sounds, so the retina is a vast bank of spatial band-pass filters, which performs Fourier analysis on retinal images.

The net effect of these band-pass filters means that the entire human visual system can be treated as a single, composite band-pass filter, which is more or less sensitive to stimuli with different spatial frequencies. The result is summarized in the form of a *contrast sensitivity function*, as in figure 3.22b, which shows that fine details at spatial frequencies greater than 30–40 cycles/degree are effectively invisible to the human eye.

Simplifications

The explanation given here (and in the next chapter) represents a simplification of the known facts. First, there's evidence that the retina contains 20 types of ganglion cells, 4 types of photoreceptors, 10 types of bipolar cells, 2 types of horizontal cells, and 30 to 40 types of amacrine cells (Kaplan 2003). Second, the idealized responses of ganglion cells presented in textbooks do not reflect the different responses observed in practice. Third, the very low firing rates referred to above rely on an assumption that ganglion cells have very high baseline firing rates, which they do not have, an issue we'll explore in the remainder of this chapter.

But just because the above account of the retina is simplified but that does not mean it is false. Indeed, science is replete with examples of how huge leaps of progress can be achieved by making use of simplifying assumptions. For example, the father of genetics, Gregor Mendel, arrived at conclusions that were essentially correct even though his simplifying

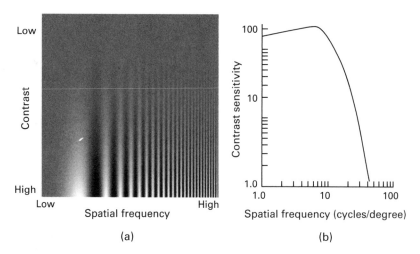

Figure 3.22

Contrast sensitivity function. (a) Sensitivity of your visual system to different spatial frequencies (stripes with different widths) is made apparent simply by looking at this figure. The height at which each stripes seems to disappear represents your threshold for seeing stripes with that particular spatial frequency. (b) Contrast sensitivity function of a typical observer. Based on Blakemore & Campbell 1969.

assumption (i.e., physical traits are inherited or not inherited in their entirety) was not.

Why Have On-Center and Off-Center Cells?

It seems a bit odd to have complementary on-center and off-center cells. Why not just have a single cell type with an output that goes above baseline when a small bright spot (surrounded by darkness) appears in the center of its receptive field and below baseline when a small dark spot (surrounded by light) appears in the center of its receptive field? The conventional reason given is that this would require the cell to have a relatively high baseline firing rate. Otherwise, if the baseline firing rate is low (as it usually is) then even a very low-contrast off-center stimulus (e.g., a not very dark spot surrounded by a not very bright annulus) would make the firing rate fall to zero. This means that a high-contrast off-center stimulus (e.g., a very dark spot against a bright background) would make the firing rate fall below zero. Well, it would, if cells could generate fewer than zero spikes per second, but they cannot. And that is the point: a cell cannot have a *negative* firing rate. But if a cell had a high baseline firing rate then it could signal the presence of a high-contrast off-center stimulus by simply reducing its firing rate, which would remain above zero. On the other hand, having a high baseline firing rate would waste energy, and neurons even at lower baseline firing rates are already expensive devices in terms of their energy consumption. Even though avoiding the need for a high baseline firing rate may be part of the reason for having on- and off-center receptive fields, there is perhaps a more important consideration that involves the notion of *linearity*.

Push-Pull Amplifiers in the Brain?
When you listen to recorded music on your iPod, CD or cassette player, or perhaps a phonograph, this involves amplifying a tiny recorded signal until it's loud enough to be heard. Although all amplifiers introduce distortions, if the one in your device is doing its job then it will keep such distortions to a minimum. But what has this to do with on-center cells?

As we have seen, the output of an on-center cell reflects the local changes in luminance of the retinal image. Ideally, this output is an undistorted representation of these changes, and as the difference between the inner and outer regions of a receptive field increases, the output of the ganglion cell increases proportionately. The key word here is "proportionately," by which I mean "linearly." In essence, if the total input (current) to a cell is represented as x and its total output (firing rate) as y then the relationship between these two is given by the generic linear equation $y = mx + c$, where m specifies how quickly the output increases with respect to the input, and c is the background or baseline firing rate (which we'll ignore for the moment). This implies that increasing the input (e.g., contrast) to a neuron by, say, 10 percent should result in a 10 percent increase in its output. A graph of output y against input x would yield a straight line with slope m, and not the S-shaped curve more typically observed in figure 3.3, which represents an input-output relationship common to many visual neurons.

Linearity is a primary consideration when passing signals around inside any system, such as an amplifier or the brain. For example, if a ganglion cell's output increased nonlinearly, say, in proportion to the *square* of the cell's input then it would be difficult for you or the brain to interpret the cell's output (i.e., $y = mx^2$). If, on the other hand, the cell's output were linearly related to its input then a doubling in the cell's output would imply a doubling in the cell's input, something easy for us, and the brain, to interpret.

More important, if the *components* of a system are linear then their outputs can be added together with the guarantee that the result is proportional to the total input to those components. Thus, if photoreceptors were linear then the total luminance within a small retinal patch would be (proportional to) the sum of photoreceptor outputs within that patch. But if the photoreceptors are *non*linear (as indeed they are) then it is a nontrivial task to work out the total luminance within a given patch of retina. For example, if a photoreceptor's output increased, say, in proportion to the square of the cell's input then you would have to find the square root of the output of every photoreceptor, and *then* add the results together to discover what the luminance within the small retinal patch was. This logic also applies to a system's composite "supercomponents," each of which consists of individual nonlinear components, such as neurons. The reason this matters is because it's usually possible to combine nonlinear components into linear composite components, as we will see shortly in the case of ganglion cells with on-center and off-center receptive fields. And if their composite components are linear then their outputs can be combined (e.g., added or subtracted) while retaining the ability to make sense of their collective outputs. Finally, the effects of random perturbations or noise on inputs can be mitigated if the distribution of that noise is known. On the other hand, if a component is *nonlinear* then its output noise distribution changes in a way that depends on the exact value of the input. This makes it extremely difficult to "undo" the effects of input noise on the outputs of a *nonlinear* component in order to estimate what the inputs were. Of course, all of these arguments apply not only to luminance, but also to *any* quantity encoded by neurons, such as contrast and line orientation.

As noted above, all amplifiers, and indeed all neurons, introduce distortions into their outputs. This is because amplifiers and neurons, though almost linear over a small, middle part of their range of output values, become *nonlinear* above and below this part. Figure 3.3 shows a typical S-shaped response curve of a neuron. The middle of this S is almost a straight line, which implies that inputs with middle values get transformed linearly (without distortion) to corresponding outputs (firing rates), whereas those with very small and very large input values undergo nonlinear transformation. Thus, as the input values increase, the corresponding outputs get squeezed into a small range of output values, and the more the input increases, the smaller this range becomes, as shown in figure 3.3.

Engineers worked out a long time ago that a linear amplifier can be made using nonlinear components provided the input signal is first split into a mostly negative and a mostly positive part, while retaining a small amount of overlap between the two parts. Next, each part is sent to a separate "subamplifier" before their outputs are recombined to yield the final amplified signal. This is true for vacuum tubes (also called "valves"), transistors, and ganglion cells. In engineering, this design is called a "class AB push-pull amplifier" because the splitting of the signal into positive and negative parts means that one half of the amplifier is "pushing" on the positive parts of the signal while the other half is "pulling" on the negative parts of the signal.

Because an off-center ganglion cell responds to a dark spot on a bright background, and an on-center ganglion cell responds to a bright spot on a dark background, these two cell types effectively split the contrast in the retinal image into "negative" and "positive" parts (review the definition of *contrast* in "Contrast" above). This is because each ganglion cell more or less "ignores" image contrasts that do not match its receptive field type, as in figures 3.23 and 3.24. If two such ganglion cells have receptive fields that cover the same region on the retina then it's as if each cell is acting like one half of a push-pull amplifier.

Now suppose a small negative contrast stimulus is presented within a small region on the retina; for example, at certain points along the dashed line in the top image in figure 3.23 or within figure 3.24. This would induce an output above baseline in the off-center ganglion cell, which would increase with the amount of negative contrast in its receptive field, as shown by the curve in figure 3.24. Unfortunately, for very small contrasts, the neuron's output is nonlinearly related to its input. The same contrast that pushes the output (firing rate) of an off-center cell above baseline inhibits the output of an on-center cell, pulling it below baseline; the output of each cell is nonlinearly related to its input contrast. Thus we have two neurons, both giving nonlinear responses to the same low-contrast stimulus, except that the off-center cell is being turned on and the on-center cell is being turned off, so their responses are in "opposite" directions. If we now subtract the response of the on-center cell from that of the off-center cell, as in figures 3.23 and 3.24 then the result is a composite transformation that has two desirable properties.

First, the *range* of contrasts over which the composite output is linear is about twice as wide as that of either neuron considered alone. Second, the transformation from retinal contrast to a composite output response is essentially *linear* for low-contrast stimuli. This is important because most parts of most retinal images we experience have low contrasts. It is worth noting that the gray levels in the middle images in figure 3.23, which represent the outputs of ganglion cells, are close to black at almost all locations in the image, which implies that the corresponding on-center

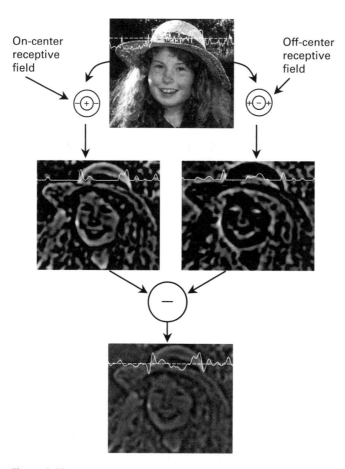

On-center receptive field

Off-center receptive field

Figure 3.23
Processing the retinal image using retinal ganglion cells with on-center and off-center receptive fields. (Top) Retinal image, with curve showing gray levels along the dashed line. This image is processed by separate populations of on-center and off-center cells. (Middle) Gray level at each point indicates the output of a cell with its receptive field centered on that point in the retinal image. (Bottom) Gray level of each point indicates the output of a hypothetical composite ganglion cell, which is the difference in the outputs of an on-center and off-center ganglion cell at corresponding positions in the images of the middle row. The curves in the middle and bottom rows show the outputs of cells at locations along the dashed line in the top image. Notice how the luminance step edges of the hat are associated with zero-crossings.

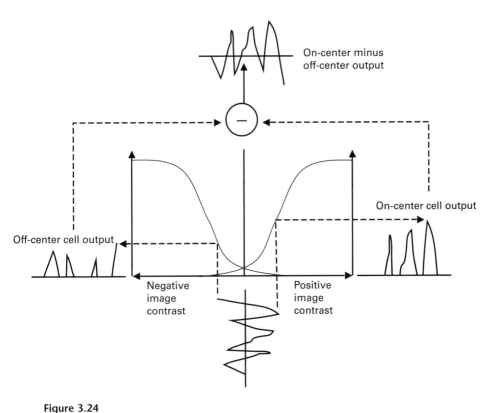

Figure 3.24
Push-pull processing using retinal ganglion cells with on-center and off-center receptive fields. The change in contrast along one line in an image (not shown) is in the bottom vertical graph. However, as each on-center cell effectively vetoes negative image contrasts, it responds only to positive contrast values. Similarly, each off-center cell effectively vetoes positive image contrasts, so it responds only to negative contrast values. Subtracting off-center cell outputs from on-center cell outputs yields the output that would be obtained from a hypothetical composite ganglion cell.

and off-center ganglion cells are effectively off at almost all locations in the image. This, in turn, implies that most of the composite ganglion cells (lower image in figure 3.23) are also off. (For display purposes, these images actually depict the logarithm of cell outputs, which exaggerates low output values.)

The upshot of all this is that we can define an "opponent pair" of on-center and off-center ganglion cells as two cells with receptive fields that cover the same circular region of the retina. We can then treat the difference between the outputs of the members of each opponent pair as if that difference is the output of a single hypothetical ganglion cell, which we will refer to as a "composite ganglion cell." This cell can have a high baseline firing rate when the contrast is zero and firing rates above baseline for positive contrasts and below baseline for negative contrasts; more importantly, its firing rate would be *linearly* related to its input over a wide range of contrast values.

Of course, if all of this applies to a pair of ganglion cells that both have a baseline firing rate at zero contrast (uniform gray) then it should also apply to a pair of cells that both have a baseline firing rate at a contrast of, say, +2, or −3, or any other contrast. In other words, the advantages of pairing up on-center and off-center cells apply not only to pairs of cells that happen to have the same baseline firing rate in response to stimuli with zero contrast but also to pairs of cells that have the same baseline firing rate in response to the same contrast, even if this contrast is highly positive or negative. By making use of such pairs of ganglion cells, increased sensitivity could be obtained all along the spectrum of contrast values.

Why Does Opponency Yield Linearity?

Although it is relatively easy to show graphically that combining the outputs of complementary neuron pairs yields a linear response (as in figures 3.23 and 3.24), the mathematical machinery that underpins all these gifts is less obvious, but goes something like this.

According to *Taylor's theorem*, any curve can be decomposed into a *constant* part, which does not vary, a *linear* part, which is a straight line, a *quadratic* part, which is bowl shaped, and so on. These "parts" are analogous to the separate components in Fourier analysis. And just as in Fourier analysis, this decomposition can be reversed, so that the original curve could be recomposed by simply adding all of these parts back together. Of course, this also applies to the curve that transforms neuronal inputs to outputs; that is, the neuronal *transfer function* shown in figure 3.24.

Taylor's theorem is not an exotic species of mathematics found in obscure academic journals, it is a cornerstone of mathematical analysis that can be found in most high school mathematics textbooks. More importantly, it can be used to show that combining the transfer functions of an on-center and an off-center ganglion cell yields a composite ganglion cell with a transfer function that is more linear than that of either ganglion cell considered in isolation, provided the transfer functions of the on-center and off-center meet two criteria. First, both transfer functions should be sufficiently smooth, as are the sigmoidal (S-shaped) transfer functions of neurons. Second, the two transfer functions should be mirror images of each other, as are those of the on-center and off-center ganglion cells. Although this second criterion is not a strict requirement for Taylor's theorem, it does guarantee that the composite transfer function is as linear as it can be for a given pair of on-center and off-center transfer functions.

If we decompose each of the two complementary transfer functions of a pair of complementary on-center and off-center cells then this is what we find: the first part (the constant) of both curves has the same value, the linear parts have the same size (magnitude) but *opposite* signs, and the quadratic parts also have the same value. More generally, *every* other part of both transfer functions has the same value (i.e., all of the terms that involve an even exponent).

Crucially, decomposing each of the on-center and off-center transfer functions into its component parts allows us to work out the effects of subtracting one transfer function from the other; all we have to do is to subtract *corresponding parts* of the two decomposed on-center and off-center transfer functions from each other. Thus, if we subtract one transfer function curve from the other, or *equivalently*, if we subtract corresponding parts of both transfer functions from each other then this is what happens. The constant parts, which are equal, cancel each other; the linear parts add together, because they have equal values but opposite signs (e.g., $x - (-x)$ = $2x$ (assuming $m = 1$ for simplicity); the quadratic parts, which are equal, also cancel each other out (e.g., $x^2 - (-x)^2 = 0$); and so on. Overall, half of the parts cancel out, leaving the remaining parts doubled in size, but otherwise unaltered. In particular, one of the parts that does not get canceled is the *linear* part, and the smoothness criterion applied above ensures that the other parts that do not get canceled out tend to be underrepresented in the original curve. Consequently, these other parts contribute very little to what is left of the composite transfer function after the two individual (on and off) transfer functions have been subtracted from each other. The result is a composite transfer function that is almost linear, and is much more linear than either of the transfer functions that made up the on- and off-center pair.

In the case of a ganglion cell, be careful not to confuse its receptive field with its transfer function. The receptive field specifies how retinal contrast at every point (photoreceptor) on the retina within that receptive field affects the total *input* to a ganglion cell (figure 3.10), whereas the transfer function defines how the total input to a ganglion cell affects its *output* firing rate (figure 3.4).

Evidence for Push-Pull Processes

The hypothetical composite ganglion cell has been introduced for purely explanatory purposes; there is no *direct* evidence for its existence (and the indirect evidence requires familiarity with terms introduced in the next chapter, so you may wish to return to this section later). However, the structure of simple cell receptive fields is consistent with a push-pull arrangement of on-center and off-center ganglion cell receptive fields (Ferster & Miller 2000; Hirsch et al. 1998; Martinez et al. 2005), which form the basis of complex and hypercomplex cells in striate cortex. For the purposes of exploring push-pull processing, it matters only that on-center and off-center ganglion cell outputs are combined at *some* point in the visual pathway. Additionally, given that simple cells receive inputs from the LGNs (lateral geniculate nuclei, which relay visual information from the retinas), we might expect simple cells to be "about as nonlinear" as LGN cells. However, in practice, the responses of simple cells are more linear than would be expected from the nonlinear responses of the LGN cells (Wielaard et al. 2001). Although this is consistent with the idea of push-pull processing (Tolhurst & Dean 1990), it has also been argued that the linear responses of simple cells is implemented through inhibitory mechanisms within striate cortex (Wielaard et al. 2001).

We should also note that linearity can also be improved by using a small amount of *negative feedback* (Regan 2000; i.e., by subtracting a small amount of output from the input), which may explain why there are connections from the cortex back to the LGNs.

More generally, it has long been recognized that certain attributes, such as color and motion, seem to operate on the basis of *opponent pairs* of cells, and the reason for this may involve the linearity such a pairing provides. Thus the aftereffects for motion (described in chapter 5) and for color (chapter 7) may be a side effect of cells that have been paired up in order to increase linearity.

As an aside, push-pull processing seems to be at work in controlling the amount of glucose in the blood. The "opposing" hormones glucagon and insulin act, respectively, to increase and to decrease blood glucose levels. As proposed by Manfred Clynes (1969), *rein control* requires the presence of two opposing hormones, and yields more robust and stable control than could be obtained with either hormone alone (Saunders, Koeslag, & Wessels 2000).

Finally, even though linearity is crucial for representing inputs accurately, there are times when it is desirable to have nonlinear transfer functions. When they are required (for example, in motion perception), these nonlinearities are not the weak affairs considered above, but are instead implemented as steplike changes in output (Heeger, Simoncelli, & Movshon 1996). Thus, even though nonlinearities in the form of S-shaped neuronal transfer functions are undesirable, their effects may be minimized by push-pull mechanisms or negative feedback. In contrast, the detection of motion (for example) may actually require the presence of sharp steplike nonlinearities, making these types of nonlinearities both desirable and necessary.

Logan's Need to Know

At the end of chapter 2, the notion that the brain acts on a "need to know" basis was discussed, and it was suggested that the eye only passes data to the brain if this data is informative about the retinal image. We have now seen that the eye passes on information about *perceptually salient features*, like luminance step edges, and that the brain can use the output of ganglion cells to identify the locations of zero-crossings that are the locations of luminance edges in the retinal image. Because different types of ganglion cells have receptive fields of different sizes, their outputs encode information about edges at different spatial scales. For example, the outputs of ganglion cells with small receptive fields reflect information regarding luminance edges that span a small image region (i.e., within a particular range of relatively high spatial frequencies), as shown in the left-hand edge map of figure 3.25c.

Crucially, a theorem by Ben Logan (1977) of Bell Laboratories suggests that the location of the luminance edges in an image provides sufficient information to reconstruct the original image at a spatial scale relevant to those edges (the word "suggests" is used here because Logan's theorem was proved for one-dimensional signals but should also apply to two-dimensional ones, like images). That is, if we know the outputs of ganglion cells then these can be used to identify the locations of zero-crossings, which correspond to edges within a particular band of spatial frequencies, and these are sufficient to reconstruct the gray levels of the image within that band of spatial frequencies. Thus, given the outputs of ganglion cells with different-sized receptive fields (which act as band-pass filters at different spatial scales), the gray levels in the retinal image are implicit in the outputs of those ganglion cells.

As we have seen in the previous section, most parts of an image do not contain edges at a spatial scale detectable by most ganglion cells' receptive fields. Consequently, for a given retinal image, most ganglion cells are

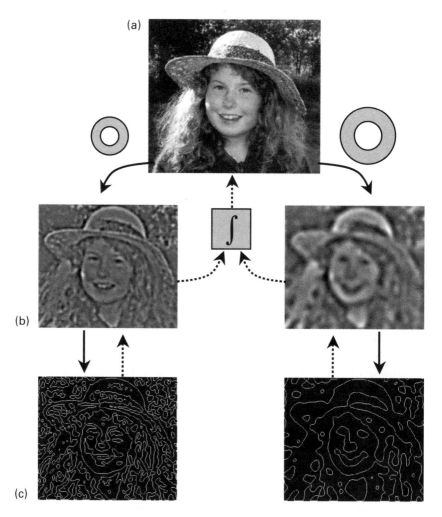

Figure 3.25

Logan's theorem. (a) Image is processed by composite ganglion cells at two spatial scales here, as indicated by the two receptive field sizes. (b) Resultant ganglion cell outputs define the location of edges, marked in (c), at a specific spatial scale. Logan's theorem suggests that knowing the locations of edges at several spatial scales, as in (c), is sufficient to be able to reconstruct the ganglion cell outputs in (b), which can be used to reconstruct the original image in (a). The dotted arrows indicate the transformations from edges to image. The outputs of on- and off-center receptive fields shown in figure 3.23 have been combined here in (b), which therefore represent the outputs of composite ganglion cells. Images produced using a computer model of ganglion cell receptive fields.

effectively off. Therefore the information received by the brain about the retinal image is conveyed by a relatively small proportion of active ganglion cells, a remarkable result given that Logan's theorem suggests that these ganglion cell outputs are sufficient to reconstruct the retinal image.

In summary, the series of transformations that begins with a retinal image and ends with a series of edge maps is reversible, as indicated by the dotted arrows in figure 3.25. Logan's theorem ensures the edge maps in figure 3.25c can be used to obtain the outputs of composite ganglion cells in figure 3.25b. Taylor's theorem guarantees that these composite ganglion cell outputs decompose into outputs of opponent pairs of on-center and off-center ganglion cell outputs. Finally, Fourier analysis means that the outputs of (composite on-center and off-center) ganglion cells with receptive fields of different sizes can be recombined to recover the original image in figure 3.25a. Collectively, these changes in the nature of representation, from retinal image to ganglion cell action potentials, correspond to mathematical transformations that provide an *efficient (re)coding* of the information implicit in the retinal image.

Receptive Fields: What Are They Good For?

As the epigraphs that open this chapter suggests, Horace Barlow seemed to recognize that the retina acts like a visual filter, discarding uninteresting data in favor of perceptually salient information. The outputs of retinal photoreceptors are not used to simply copy the retinal image verbatim onto a sheet of corresponding neurons deep inside the brain, where a *homunculus* (little man) looks at it and tells the brain what the image contains. Indeed, this could not be the case because the outputs of retinal photoreceptors never reach the brain intact. They are first "distorted" by being filtered through an array of ganglion cells. These cells provide the brain with signals that are very different from the photograph-like image in figure 2.13 captured by the outputs of retinal photoreceptors. However, even though the action potentials streaming along the axons of ganglion cells bear no obvious resemblance to the retinal image, Logan's theorem suggests that the information these spikes convey is sufficient to reconstruct the entire image—given the right machinery.

In essence, the retinal ganglion cells' outputs represent a specific method for encoding the retinal image. From a purely intuitive viewpoint, this encoding seems to be doing the right things, like signaling the presence of changes in image luminance and ignoring uniformly lit regions. But, aside from this reassuring observation, how do we know that the representation implied by the outputs of retinal ganglion cells is a good representation of the image? If, by "good," we mean an encoding that preserves most of the information in the retinal image then a good representation would be an "information-preserving" representation. But how could we tell if a representation preserves information? Well, as a first guess, if we could measure the amount of information in the image and compare it to the amount of information in the collective spike trains of ganglion cells then we would know how much information about the image was preserved by ganglion cell outputs. This problem has been tackled by a number of researchers, who arrived at the following conclusion.

Under good lighting conditions, the way to maximize the amount of information about the retinal image in ganglion cell outputs is for ganglion cells to have Mexican hat receptive fields. In fact, Logan's theorem strongly suggests that the transformation provided by human retinal ganglion cells and horseshoe crab photoreceptors preserves almost all of the information implicit in the retinal image. Thus, in terms of Marr's computational framework, the task performed by both visual systems involves preserving information about the retinal image (even if that occasionally produces the wrong result, as exemplified by the Chevreul illusion). Notice that preserving information is achieved by recoding the image data into a relatively compact representation. A set of related ideas has been proposed to account for this, and because they all yield an efficient coding of the retinal image, it goes under the name of the "efficient coding hypothesis."

In 1982, Mandyam Srinivasan, Simon Laughlin, and Andreas Dubs published a paper that showed that the way for cells in the fly's brain to maximize the amount of information they transmit about the "retinal" image under poor lighting conditions is for receptive fields to be less like a Mexican hat and more like a flat tortilla. This was followed in the early 1990s by a series of key theoretical papers, principally by Hans van Hateren (1992) and by Joseph Atick and A. Norman Redlich (1990, 1992) on redundancy reduction and neuronal function (see "A Bit of the Hard Stuff," below).

From Mexican Hats to Bells

Most parts of the physical world vary smoothly from place to place, so that most parts of an image also tend to vary smoothly from place to place. Of course, we are surrounded by exceptions to this observation, but from a purely statistical viewpoint, the number of places where the world varies continuously far outnumber the number of places where it undergoes step changes; and so it is for the retinal images derived from such a world. For example, adjacent parts on the surface of a leaf are about the same color and texture almost everywhere. On a larger scale, adjacent parts of a river surface tend to be similar. These are just different ways of saying that, because adjacent parts of the world have similar physical properties, adjacent parts of an image tend to have similar visual properties, such as color and texture. More important, these are just informal ways of saying that adjacent parts of an image are *correlated*. Sending the raw output of each photoreceptor to the brain would therefore result in a huge duplication of labor because almost every photoreceptor would have an output that is, to all intents and purposes, indistinguishable from that of its neighbors. As we have already observed, a ganglion cell will not even get out of bed unless adjacent photoreceptors within its receptive field have different outputs (e.g., unless the receptive field lies across a step edge in image luminance).

If each receptive field was structured so that its ganglion cell output was just the average output of the photoreceptors in that receptive field then nearby ganglion cells would have very similar (correlated) outputs. Given that sending correlated signals to the brain is clearly a bad idea, what would be an efficient scheme for information transmission? Well, at the other extreme from sending correlated signals, an obvious alternative would be to ensure that nearby ganglion cells sent only unique or *un*correlated signals to the brain. It turns out that the Mexican hat structure ensures not only that interesting parts of the image, such as edges, yield a change in ganglion cell output, but also that ganglion cells with neighboring receptive fields have outputs that are largely uncorrelated (Nirenberg et al. 2001). Thus the Mexican hat receptive fields essentially *de*correlate the correlated inputs they receive from neighboring photoreceptors. In contrast to early reports (Hartline & Ratliff 1958) of the Mexican hat structure, which stressed its ability to exaggerate step edges in luminance, modern accounts increasingly consider this to be a side effect of retinal neuronal machinery transmitting as much information as possible to the brain.

Although the information-theoretic account of receptive field structure is satisfying, it seems at odds with the following intriguing observation: if the brightness of the retinal image is reduced by simply dimming the lights in a room then the Mexican hat receptive field structure gradually transforms into a simple bump (more precisely, the classic bell-shaped curve). In other words, under poor lighting conditions, all of the photoreceptors in the on-center receptive field of a ganglion cell have an excitatory effect, but those near to the center of the receptive field are more excitatory than those at the periphery (and the converse is applies to off-center receptive fields). Consequently, the retinal ganglion cell's output is approximately proportional to the mean output of the photoreceptors in its receptive field. As discussed above, this seems to be a very poor scheme because it seems to imply that the outputs of nearby ganglion cells would be correlated. However, under low lighting conditions, this actually ensures that as much information as possible is transmitted. The reason is the arch enemy of all system designers (including evolution): noise.

Most images consist of big, blocky structures, like trees and furniture, plus relatively small structures, like bark and texture, which correspond to low and high spatial frequencies, respectively. Because image noise consists of stray photons of light and jitter within individual photoreceptors, it tends to affect the activity of individual photoreceptors, and therefore to preferentially disrupt the representation of smaller visual structures, rather than the big blocky structures. As if this weren't bad enough, natural images tend to have almost all their contrast associated with the big, blocky structures, rather than relatively small visual structures. So only a small proportion of the contrast in images comes from its fine details, and most image noise tends to exist at the level of these fine details.

Although the amount of image noise is pretty much constant, under low-light conditions, the impact of the retinal image on photoreceptor outputs necessarily decreases, which suggests that the *proportion* of noise in the photoreceptor outputs must increase. In the limiting case of very low light levels, almost all of the photoreceptor outputs are caused by noise, rather than by elements of the image.

A practical way of reducing the effects of image noise is to take a simple average of the outputs of a set of neighboring photoreceptors. Because noise varies randomly around a mean value, when all the photoreceptor outputs (which include noise) are added up, all the parts of the image noise below the mean tend to cancel out all the parts of the noise above the mean. Under low-light conditions, the way to maximize the information about the image is to ensure a ganglion cell's output is a particular weighted average of the outputs of photoreceptors in its receptive field. This weighted average can be realized in the form of a receptive field that is not a Mexican hat, but a simple bump (the bell-shaped curve). Indeed, experimental observations confirm that this is what happens to the structure of ganglion cell receptive fields under low-light conditions (Kuffler 1953; Barlow, Fitzhugh, & Kuffler 1957; but also see Duffy & Hubel 2007). Even though such a receptive field structure tends to increase the correlation between nearby ganglion cell outputs, this is more than offset by the reduction in the amount of image noise transmitted by ganglion cell outputs, so that there is a net *increase* in the information transmitted about the retinal image to the brain (Attick and Redlich 1990).

A Bit of the Hard Stuff

As is almost always the case with scientific phenomena, scientists have proposed several competing hypotheses to explain the structure of receptive fields: redundancy reduction (Atick & Redlich 1992; Nadal & Parga 1993); predictive coding (Rao & Ballard 1999; Srinavasen, Laughlin, & Dubs 1982); maximizing sparseness (Foldiak & Young 1995); minimizing energy (Niven, Anderson, & Laughlin 2007); independent component analysis (Bell & Sejnowski 1995; Stone 2004); and efficient coding (Atick, Li, & Redlich 1992; Attneave 1954; Barlow 1961; Laughlin 1981). These hypotheses make use of different, but related, general principles to predict receptive field structure, and each hypothesis generates similar (but not identical) predictions regarding the structure of receptive fields. This is interesting because the conservative nature of evolution suggests that it is likely that a single general principle is used to encode retinal images. If so, then this general principle may also apply throughout the brain, or at least to its other sensory modalities, such as hearing and touch. In other words, the principles used to encode retinal images may apply throughout the brain and may therefore represent the "holy grail" of brain function.

Even though these related hypotheses are undeniably elegant, elegance is not scientific evidence. But there is a growing body of evidence in support of the general idea that neurons act as efficient information channels, consistent with the efficient coding hypothesis. Specifically, pairs of cells that are neighbors within several brain regions have been shown to have outputs that are uncorrelated, even though they probably receive similar (correlated) inputs. Thus, cells within the retina (ganglion cells; Nirenberg et al. 1991), simple cells in striate cortex (Ecker et al. 2010), and cells in inferotemporal cortex (Gawne & Richmond 1993) may act as efficient information channels by minimizing the extent to which each cell's output overlaps with that of its neighbors.

At present, most of these hypotheses give a reasonably good account of the experimental findings and are therefore difficult to tease apart. But we have at least moved away from the hand-waving theories that seem, in retrospect, to be the equivalent of plausible but vague just-so stories. Now the first step of formulating rigorous, and therefore testable, hypotheses has been taken, it is only a matter of time before we discover which of the general principles implicit in the above theories underpins the neuronal coding of retinal images.

The Efficient Coding Hypothesis

The various principles mentioned above can be conveniently classified as variants on the central theme of the efficient coding hypothesis. In essence, the efficient coding hypothesis states that neurons should encode sensory inputs as efficiently as possible, where efficiency is measured in terms of Shannon information (see chapter 7). The formalization of information was first described in 1948 as part of Shannon and Weaver's information theory (Shannon 1948; Shannon and Weaver 1949), which sparked a huge amount of research in perceptual psychology in the 1950s. In particular, Barlow (1961) and Attneave (1954) applied information theory to the problems of perception, and their ideas underpin the modern incarnation of the efficient coding hypothesis (e.g., Simoncelli 2003); an idea which we will revisit many times throughout the remainder of this book.

4   The Visual Brain

Other maps are such shapes with their islands and capes!
But we've got our brave captain to thank:
(So the crew would protest) "that he's bought us the best—
A perfect and absolute blank!"
—Lewis Carroll, *The Hunting of the Snark*

Impressions

Drunk on information, spikes tumble into cortical space.

Visual information is processed in the *visual* or *occipital cortex*, which lies at the back of the brain, as shown in figure 4.1 (plate 5). Within the visual cortex, several distinct regions provide increasingly specialized forms of processing. The *striate* or *primary visual cortex* (V1) seems to act as a visual manager, parceling out different types of visual information to specialized parts within the *secondary visual cortex* (V2). As we will see below, this process of specialization seems to continue in brain regions more distant from striate cortex.

The basic properties of neurons in the visual cortex were discovered by David Hubel and Torsten Wiesel, for which they received the 1981 Nobel Prize. Hubel (1988) describes how, in 1958 and as part of their normal experimental procedure, they had connected the output of a recording electrode to an audio amplifier, so that every action potential from a single neuron in striate cortex was heard as a loud click:

The position of the microelectrode tip was unusually stable, so that we were able to listen to one cell for about nine hours. We tried everything short of standing on our heads to get it to fire. After some hours we began to have a vague feeling that shining light on one particular part of the retina was evoking some response, so we tried concentrating our efforts there. To stimulate, we used mostly white circular

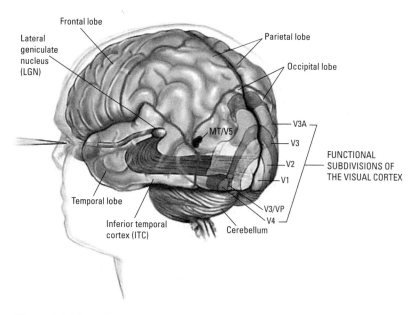

Lateral geniculate nucleus (LGN)

Frontal lobe

Parietal lobe

Occipital lobe

V3A

V3

MT/V5

V2

V1

FUNCTIONAL
SUBDIVISIONS OF
THE VISUAL CORTEX

Temporal lobe

Inferior temporal cortex (ITC)

V3/VP

V4

Cerebellum

Figure 4.1 (plate 5)
Major divisions of the human brain and visual cortex. Reproduced with permission, copyright © 1999 Terese Winslow.

spots and black spots. For black spots we would take a 1 by 2 inch glass laboratory slide, onto which we glued a black spot, and shove it into a slot in an optical instrument to project onto the retina. For white spots, we used a slide made of brass with a hole drilled in it. After about five hours of struggle, we suddenly had the impression that the glass with the dot was occasionally producing a response, but the response seemed to have little to do with the dot. Eventually, we caught on: it was the sharp but faint shadow cast by the glass as we slid it into the slot that was doing the trick. Most amazing was the contrast between the machine-gun discharge when the orientation of the stimulus was just right, and the utter lack of a response if we changed the orientation or simply shone a bright flashlight into the cat's eyes.

Clearly, from Hubel's account, he and Wiesel expected cortical cells to have center-surround receptive fields like those of retinal ganglion cells. Instead, they discovered that cells in striate cortex seemed to respond to elongated edges.

Their discovery was a crucial step in understanding human vision because it suggested that the outputs of ganglion cells could be combined to produce cells with more complex receptive fields. More important, it implied the possibility of a visual hierarchy of increasingly complex receptive fields, with increasingly complex functions. In the fifty years since then, researchers have discovered cells that respond not only to edges (as above) but also to color, depth, curvature, hands, objects, people walking, faces, and even specific individuals. But we have leapt ahead too far in our account of the history of vision. To fully appreciate the momentous progress made since 1958, we need to back up and consider the basic neuroanatomy of the visual system.

From Retina to Visual Cortex

At about the time Hubel and Wiesel were probing cells in the striate cortex of the cat, Jerome Lettvin and colleagues (1959) discovered cells that seemed to respond to even more complex visual features than edges—in the retina of a frog. Neurons, known as "bug detectors," that respond almost exclusively to the erratic motion of a fly are not synthesized in the brain from the outputs of lowly center-surround ganglion cells, but *are* retinal ganglion cells (Lettvin et al. 1959). Indeed, most of the computational machinery responsible for vision in the frog resides in the retina. Similarly, the computational machinery that allows a rabbit to detect the motion of a fox is located not in the rabbit's cortex but in its retina. For these, relatively primitive species, the eye does not send "raw" luminance or contrast information to the brain, where it's analyzed for the presence of flies or foxes. Indeed, it seems to be a rule of thumb that the relative amounts of computational load carried by the retina versus the brain increase as we descend the evolutionary tree. Or, as Denis Baylor of Stanford Medical School put it, "The dumber the animal, the smarter the retina" (Baylor in Montgomery 1995).

The discovery that retinal ganglion cells have center-surround receptive fields in humans might suggest that the human brain delays detailed analysis of the retinal image until after the information has left the retina via the optic nerve. While this is true, it is not the whole truth. Specifically, while complex structural features of the retinal image are the province of the cortex in humans, the decomposition of the retinal image into key components, such as color and motion, begins at the retina. More importantly, the manner in which the different components of the retinal image are encoded by retinal neurons places constraints on the overall computational architecture of different cortical regions. The division of labor that begins at the retina defines two distinct processing streams (the M and P streams), which remain separate, at least to some extent, after they have reached the cortex.

From Retina to LGN

As described in chapter 2, each of the one million retinal ganglion cells in the retina sends a single axon out of the back of the retina via the optic disc (blind spot), and these fibers collectively form the *optic nerve* (see figures 2.10 and 2.11). The relatively well organized spatial arrangement of ganglion cells quickly breaks down within the optic nerve, which is just a bundle of tangled axons. When the optic nerve from each eye reaches the *optic chiasm*, half the fibers cross to the other side of the brain (the chiasm is named after the Greek letter chi [χ] to denote the crossing point). Specifically, half the fibers from the innermost or *nasal* part of each retina cross over to the other half of the brain, whereas those on the outermost or *temporal* part do not, as shown in figure 4.2.

The left-right reversal imposed by the process of forming an image on the retina ensures that the entire right side of the scene, called the "right visual hemifield," ends up on the left side of each retina, and vice versa for the "left visual hemifield," as shown in figure 4.2. Thus information about the right side of the visual field ends up on the left side of both retinal images. So, if the brain wants to keep all the information about the right side of the visual field together, it can do one of two things: (1) make information from the left side of the left retinal image cross over to join information from the left side of the right retina; or (2) make information from the left side of the right retinal image cross over to join information from the left side of the left retina (of course, a similar logic also applies to the left side of the visual field). In fact, the chiasm seems to follow option 2, perhaps because this involves shorter axons, and therefore less delay, than option 1. After the optic chiasm, each newly formed bundle of axons collectively constitutes an *optic tract*; each carries all the information from both retinas about the same half of the visual field.

Each optic tract terminates at the first synapses after the retina, within one of a pair of six-layered structures called the "lateral geniculate nuclei" (LGNs; from Latin *geniculatus* for "bent like a knee"). Each of the six layers within one LGN represents the scene of one visual hemifield. For example, within the left LGN, each layer represents information from the left half of both retinas, which corresponds to the scene in the right visual hemifield. In practice, separate types of ganglion cells carry information regarding different aspects of the retinal image, and are segregated into distinct layers within the LGN, with each ganglion cell delivering its output to only one layer (figure 4.3). If the ganglion cell axons from the left half of each retina behaved like simple light guides then their outputs would form an image of the scene in the right visual hemifield within *each* layer of the LGN. In other words, the spatial layout of ganglion cells in each retina is

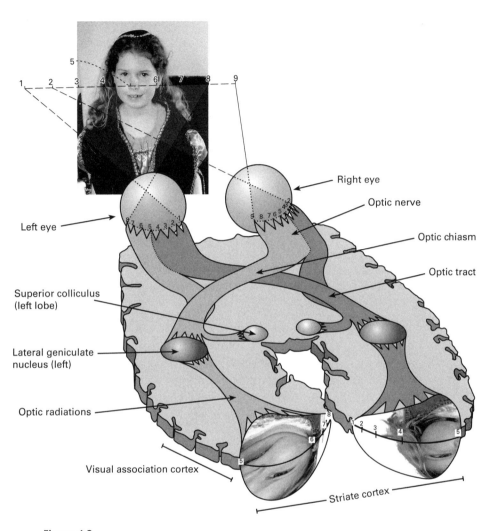

Figure 4.2
How the visual world gets transformed by the pathways of the visual system. Modified from Frisby & Stone 2010.

reflected in the layout of their terminating axons within the LGN, which define a *retinotopic* or *topographic* map within each layer of the LGN.

The layers of each LGN lie on top of one another, and are "in register," so that the points encountered by a needle driven down through the six layers would correspond to the same point in the visual field. If a needle were to be driven down through the left LGN, along the dashed line in figure 4.3a, then it would encounter information from the left half retinas

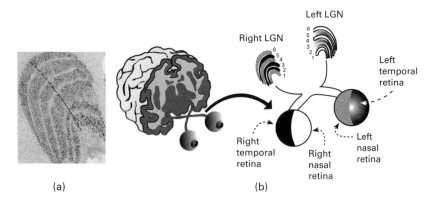

Figure 4.3
Lateral geniculate nuclei (LGNs). (a) Cross section of the lateral geniculate nucleus, with the magnocellular layers 1 and 2 at the base and the parvocellular layers 3–6 at the top. Reproduced with permission. (b) Schematic diagram showing the anatomical origins of each layer in the LGNs. From Frisby & Stone 2010.

of the left and right eyes in this order: R, L, R, L, L, R. Rather than using the labels L and R, a more general terminology is *ipsilateral* and *contralateral*, which specifies whether a given layer receives projections from the eye that is on the same side as the LGN under consideration or on the opposite side, as shown in figure 4.3a. No one knows why the layers are arranged in this order, nor why there is a reversal in the sequence between layers 4 and 5. Hypothesizing that this reversal is there just to make the sequence harder to remember, Hubel (1988) has declared that "we really have no idea why there is a sequence at all."

All cells in the LGNs have on-center or off-center receptive fields that differ little from the ganglion cells that provide their input, and in certain species (mink, ferret, and possibly monkey), the on- and off-center cells innervate separate layers within the LGNs. No one knows why the LGNs appear to act as a simple relay station, which apparently adds little or nothing to the processing of retinal information. Indeed, Andrew Derrington (2001) has described the LGNs as "a huge embarrassment to visual neuroscientists."

Magno, Parvo, and Konio Layers in the LGNs
Even to the naked eye, it's apparent that the LGNs consist of layers, as shown in figure 4.3a. If we consider pairs of corresponding layers *across* the left and right LGNs, then each pair receives information from opposite visual hemifields. So layers in the left LGN receive information from the

left (L) and right (R) retinas in this order: R, L, R, L, L, R, whereas corresponding layers in the right LGN receive information from the retinas in the opposite order: L, R, L, R, R, L.

The two lower *magnocellular* layers (1–2) are populated by large cells (*magnus* is Latin for "large"). Within the left LGN, magnocellular layer 1 receives input from the right eye, whereas magnocellular layer 2 receives input from the left eye. Each magnocellular layer receives the outputs of *parasol retinal ganglion cells*. These ganglion cells make up about 10 percent of the total. Because they receive most of their inputs from a relatively large number of rods, they have large receptive fields (6–8 times as large as cells in the parvocellular layers, described below). Their dependence on rod-mediated vision means that they, and the LGN cells they innervate, have transient responses to low-luminance stimuli; they're thought to encode motion-related information, as well as achromatic (black and white) contrast. These parasol retinal ganglion cells and the magnocellular LGN layers they innervate constitute the start of the magno (M) processing stream.

In contrast, the four upper *parvocellular* layers (3–6) of the LGNs are populated by tiny cells (*parvus* is Latin for "small"). These four parvocellular layers receive the outputs of *midget retinal ganglion cells*, which make up about 80 percent of all ganglion cells in the retina. These ganglion cells receive their inputs from a small number of cone receptors, and therefore have small receptive fields, which respond to color and are believed to mediate responses to red/green contrasts. They also have a weak response to achromatic contrast and are thought to be involved in encoding static form. Recall that, within the left LGN, layer 3 receives inputs from the left eye, whereas layer 4 receives inputs from the right eye. These midget retinal ganglion cells and the parvocellular LGN layers they innervate constitute the start of the parvo (P) processing stream.

Finally, there are the *konio* layers, a relatively recent discovery. At the base of each parvocellular and magnocellular layer, a thinner konio layer receives inputs from *bistratified* retinal ganglion cells, which constitute less than 10 percent of all ganglion cells. Bistratified cells respond to blue light by increasing their firing rate, and to yellow light by decreasing their firing rate (other cells seem to display the opposite responses to blue and yellow, but more on this color opponency in chapter 7).

The confusing anatomical arrangement of the retino-geniculate pathway has two consequences. The first is that information about the left side of the viewed scene is kept together within the brain, despite the fact that this information is initially recorded as the right half-image of the two eyes (and vice versa for the right visual field). The second consequence is that the different types of information encoded by different classes of ganglion cells are kept separate, although the precise nature of the information encoded in each layer remains a topic of research.

This division of labor between different types of ganglion cells, LGN layers, and especially between the magnocellular and parvocellular sets of LGN layers is thought to underpin separate processing streams that reach far into the cortex. In essence, the magnocellular (M) stream is involved in motion detection and analysis, whereas the parvocellular (P) stream is involved in color and form analysis.

From LGN to Striate Cortex

The *neocortex* is sheet of neurons, a 1.7 mm thick and 1,300 square centimeters (cm^2) in area, that constitutes the outermost part of the two *cerebral hemispheres* of the brain. Every cubic millimeter of neocortex contains 100,000 neurons, and the whole neocortex contains a total of approximately 25 billion neurons, each of which receives inputs via 4,000 synapses.

The global structure of the visual cortex is organized *retinotopically*; that is, adjacent points in the retinal image usually project to adjacent points in striate cortex, as shown in figure.4.4. Note that the central foveal region

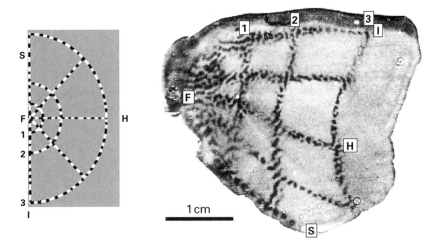

Figure 4.4

Macaque monkey striate cortex (right) showing activity evoked by visual stimulus (left). Corresponding regions in the visual field and the visual cortex are indicated by letters and numbers: S = superior (upper) visual field; F = fovea; I = inferior (lower) visual field; H = horizontal meridian. Reproduced with modifications from Tootell et al. 1988.

of the retina projects to a relatively large area in the LGNs and striate cortex. The disproportionate allocation of cortical space to the fovea reflects the dense packing of cones in the fovea, as well as the relatively large amount of neuronal processing allocated to the central part of the retinal image.

The visual cortex is organized into six distinct layers, numbered from 1 to 6, with layer 1 at the surface, as shown in figure 4.5. Cells within the LGNs send their axons to the primary visual or striate cortex, which derives its name from the stripe that runs along layer 4 where the axons from the LGNs terminate. Because these axons innervate (project to) only primary visual cortex, the sudden disappearance of this stripe marks the border between primary visual cortex (V1) and secondary visual cortex (V2), as shown in figure 4.6. This stripe, called the "stria of Gennari," was first observed by Francesco Gennari in 1776 (*stria* is Latin for "fine streak").

The division of labor that began with the different types of photoreceptors and continued with the retinal ganglion cells and the LGNs extends

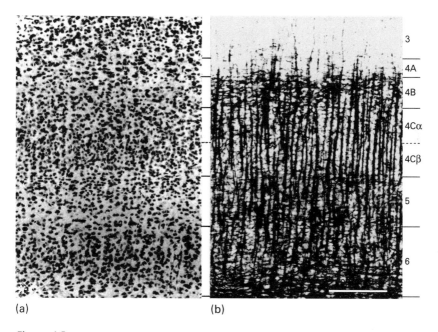

(a)   (b)

Figure 4.5
Monkey striate cortex. Microscopic enlargements of sections stained to emphasize cell bodies in (a) and nerve fibers in (b). The numbers at the right refer to various layers that can be distinguished microscopically. Courtesy LeVay, Hubel, and Wiesel (1975).

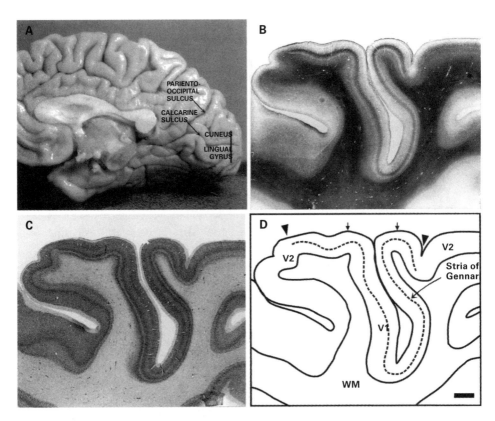

Figure 4.6
Striate cortex (V1) as defined by the stria of Gennari. (A) Photograph of the medial
(inner) surface of the human occipital lobe. (B) Photomicrograph of a cross section
through the occipital lobe, stained for myelin. (C) Prominent cell-dense layers that
distinguish striate cortex. (D) Extent of striate cortex (arrowheads) was determined
by tracing the stria (dashed line) in the myelin-stained section. Scale bar: 2 mm.
Reproduced with permission from Andrews, Halpern, & Purvis 1997.

into the primary visual cortex. Specifically, the projections of the magnocellular LGN layers terminate in a sublayer of layer 4 (4Cα), whereas
projections of the parvocellular LGN layers terminate in sublayer (4Cβ),
as shown in figure 4.7. Collaterals (subbranches) of the axons from
cells in the LGN also innervate the pyramidal cells in cortical layer 6,
which send projections back to the LGN cells that innervate them. There
is thus a complete, and quite specific, set of feedback connections from
striate cortex to LGNs. Indeed, most of the input connections to the
LGN come, not from the retina, but from these V1 feedback connections.

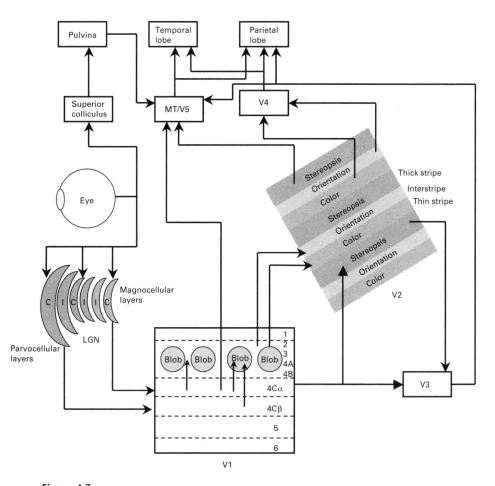

Figure 4.7
Unpacking the striate cortex. The outputs of different ganglion cells in each eye project to specific layers of the LGNs (C = contralateral, I = ipsilateral). These then project to striate cortex (V1), which project to discrete stripes of V2. These project to areas V3–V5, which are specialized for processing different types of information.

The function of these connections is not known, but interfering with them seems to decrease the specificity of LGN cells. To continue the theme of linearity introduced at the end of chapter 3, another possibility is that the LGN–striate system is made more linear by using feedback from striate cortex to LGNs, which may explain why striate cortex projects to the LGNs.

Simple Cells

As described by David Hubel in the introduction to this chapter, he and Torsten Wiesel were the first to discover cells in striate cortex that responded to elongated strips of contrast in the form of either a line or luminance edge, which they named "simple cells," shown in figures 4.8 and 4.9 (plate 6). The elongated structure of each simple cell receptive field makes it sensitive to the precise orientation of lines on the retina, known as its "preferred orientation," shown in figure 4.10.

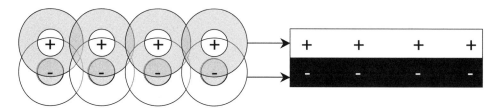

Figure 4.8
Combining the outputs from LGN cells with center-surround receptive fields to create a simple cell receptive field that responds best to a luminance step edge at one (horizontal) *preferred orientation*. The sign (+,–) indicates whether light has an excitatory or inhibitory effect on a cell within each region of its receptive field.

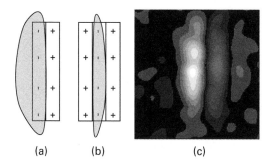

Figure 4.9 (plate 6)
(a–b) Schematic receptive fields of simple cells found in primary visual cortex, with shaded regions showing the approximate pattern of light and dark that yields the maximum response from each cell. The sign (+,–) indicates whether light has an excitatory or inhibitory effect on the simple cell within each region of its receptive field. The two basic types of simple cells are sensitive to (a) luminance edges and (b) lines. Receptive fields with the + and – signs swapped also exist in equal numbers. (c) Color-coded response of a simple cell receptive field, with red showing inhibitory region, and green showing excitatory region. Reproduced with permission.

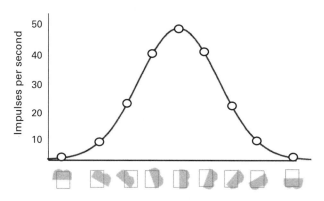

Figure 4.10
Schematic orientation tuning curve of a simple cell with a vertical preferred orientation. From Frisby & Stone 2010.

Because simple cells receive inputs from LGN cells with center-surround receptive fields, it seemed natural to suppose that the outputs of LGN cells are combined to synthesize the elongated structure of a typical simple cell receptive field, as shown in figure 4.8. Indeed, researchers have found that the excitatory elongated region of a simple cell's receptive field corresponds to the excitatory centers of on-center LGN receptive field cells, whereas the inhibitory elongated region corresponds to the inhibitory centers of off-center LGN cells. This supports the hypothesis that a simple cell's receptive field is the result of a reasonably straightforward integration of on- and off-center receptive field cells. The width of a simple cell's receptive field determines whether it responds to narrow or gradual changes in luminance (i.e., sharp or blurred luminance edges), which in turn is determined by the size of its constituent LGN receptive fields, as shown in figure 4.8. That LGN cells have receptive fields with specific sizes on the retina implies that each simple cell has not only a preferred orientation but also a *preferred width*. Specifically, each simple cell responds best to either sharp or gradual changes in luminance, which correspond to high and low spatial frequencies, respectively. Each simple cell may combine the outputs of its constituent LGN cells outputs using the push-pull design principle described in chapter 3, which may account for the linear responses of simple cells to increasing contrast (Heeger 1991).

When Hubel and Wiesel drove an electrode vertically downward from the cortical surface, they found that the cells that responded best to lines and edges were within layers 3, 4, and 6 (figure 4.5). Moreover, they found

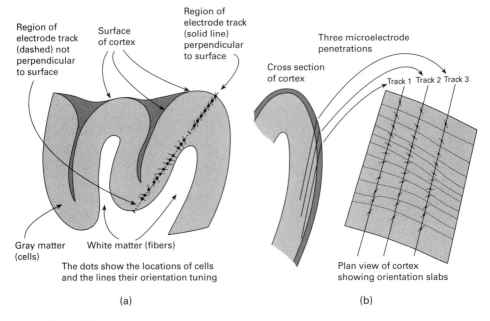

Figure 4.11
Results from microelectrode penetrations revealing orientation-tuned columns in striate cortex. Adapted from Hubel 1981; reproduced from Frisby & Stone 2010.

that all the orientation-sensitive cells encountered within a single vertical needle penetration responded to the *same* line orientation, as shown in figure 4.11a. Vernon Mountcastle (1957) discovered this organization into *columns* in other brain regions, and it was soon established that the striate cortex is organized along similar lines.

As Hubel (1988) would say in 1982, this probing in different directions yielded major new insights into the structure of the visual cortex: "I think that the most important advance was the strategy of making long microelectrode penetrations through the cortex, recording from cell after cell, comparing responses to natural stimuli, with the object not only of finding the optimal stimulus for particular cells, but also of learning what the cells had in common and how they were grouped." The result of such probing showed that the line orientation encoded by different columns changed gradually across the cortex, but with occasional "jumps" in orientation (which were later discovered to be associated with *orientation singularities*; see "The packing problem" below). Thus, even though the cortex has a finite thickness, and therefore has three dimensions, by forcing all simple cells within a single column to respond to the same orientation, the brain sacrifices one dimension for representing different orientations and effectively treats the neocortex as a two-dimensional sheet. It later became apparent that these orientation singularities usually contain cells that are insensitive to orientation, but sensitive to color. As such, they were labeled "color blobs."

Just as the outputs of cells with center-surround receptive fields can yield simple cell receptive fields, so the outputs of simple cells can feed into cells that have more complex receptive fields, known as "complex cells." These cells reside within layers 2, 3, 5, and 6, with simple cells restricted to the upper part of layer 4. Among the most common of these are cells that respond best to motion in a specific direction, known as the cell's "preferred direction," and to a specific speed, known as its "preferred speed." Complex cells also respond to the same edge stimuli as simple cells at a single orientation, but over a range of retinal positions and to both positive and negative contrasts (Gawne 2000). Complex cells that can be used to construct receptive fields with even more complex structures are known as "hypercomplex cells." In principle, the push-pull design (proposed for ganglion cells in chapter 3) may also apply to pairs of simple cells that contribute to each complex cell, although there is, as yet, no reported evidence for this.

Temporal Receptive Fields

We already know that the receptive field of a simple cell has a spatial structure defined over a small region on the retina. But that field also has a *temporal structure* defined over a small interval of time following the onset of a stimulus. In other words, the response of a simple cell varies over time after the onset of a particular stimulus in a characteristic manner; just like the ringing of a wine glass after it has been tapped.

The particular way in which the cell's response changes after stimulus onset defines the temporal structure of its receptive field. Moreover, just as each cell has a preferred spatial frequency (e.g., bar width), so it also has a preferred *temporal* frequency, which determines how quickly a stimulus has to change in order to stimulate a given cell (e.g., a series of bars like those in figure 3.16b, moving across the retina). Because these retinal changes over time are usually caused by something moving across the retina, these cells effectively signal the presence of such movement. As each cell only responds to motion of a particular spatial pattern, there exists a *spatiotemporal* stimulus that evokes the best response from each cell, and that stimulus is usually the one that matches the spatiotemporal structure of the cell's receptive field.

Maps in Primary Visual Cortex

As described in Hubel's 1988 account quoted above, the response properties of a given cell were established by presenting a line to the eyes, and
adjusting its orientation and position in order to elicit a response. Hubel
and Wiesel found that stimulating, say, the left eye gave a larger response
than the right eye, but if they advanced the electrode by about 0.5 mm
across the cortex, then the converse was true. By coloring each point on
the striate cortex in black or white in accordance with the (left or right)
eye that projected to each point, they were able to construct an ocularity
map, as shown in figure 4.13. Even though most simple cells were *binocular*, and therefore responded to stimulation from both eyes, the degree of
ocular dominance gradually shifted as they advanced the electrode by a few
millimeters across the cortex. It thus seemed as if the eye-specific responses
of LGN cells were reflected in the cortex, with adjacent regions flip-flopping
between the eyes. These early discoveries by Hubel and Wiesel and others
were later confirmed, using techniques that allowed images of whole areas
of cortex to be captured, resulting in whole series of beautiful color-coded
orientation maps (figure 4.12, plate 7), direction maps, color maps, and
ocularity maps (figure 4.13).

Hypercolumns

To detect a line of any orientation within any region of the retinal image,
the brain must have a "complete set" of simple cells that have preferred
orientations that span the range from 0 to 180 degrees for every small
patch of the retinal image. If the brain did not have cells with a preferred
orienation of, say, 90 degrees (i.e., vertical) within one patch of retina then
we'd be unable to see vertical lines within that patch. Such a hypothetical
complete set is known as an "orientation hypercolumn."

More generally, to detect a line of any orientation, any color, and any
width, moving in any direction and at any speed within any region of the
retinal image, the brain must have a "complete set" of cells for every small
patch of the retinal image. In other words, it must have a set of cells that
can detect all line orientations, widths, directions, speeds, and color, and
this set must be reduplicated thousands of times across the striate cortex.
Such a complete set or complex hypercolumn is a hypothetical entity that
includes the orientation hypercolumn defined above. An example of a
simplified hypercolumn that can detect only orientation, size, and ocularity is shown in the diagram at the top of figure 4.14. Notice how different
simple cell receptive field types pick out different types of image features.
For example, the wide vertical stripes on the zebra's body are apparent

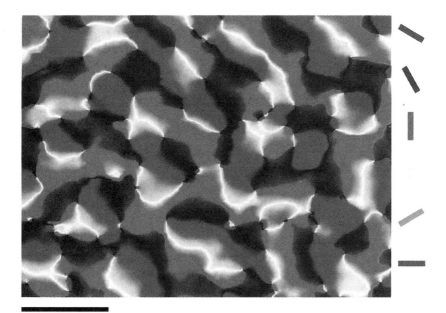

Figure 4.12 (plate 7)
False-color orientation map in primary visual cortex, as viewed from above the cortical surface. The preferred orientation of cells within each cortical area is indicated
by color, as shown in the key on the right of the figure. Scale bar: 1 mm. Reproduced
with permission from Blasdel 1992.

mainly in the outputs of simple cells with large, vertically oriented receptive fields, as shown in the middle right-hand panel. Thus each small patch
in the retinal image is analyzed by a complete set of receptive field types.
The model shown here has simple cells with receptive fields at two orientations and three spatial scales, making a total of six types. The corresponding "hypercolumn" of six simple cell types would be located in a small
region of striate cortex. So, if each simple cell type defined a single column,
then this hypothetical hypercolumn would consist of six columns.

Pictures in the Head?
The various maps discovered in the visual cortex confirmed that the retinal
image really does not give rise to anything that resembles a "picture in
the head." Indeed, the "picture in the head" within striate cortex looks
nothing like that retinal image, with different properties represented by
different subpopulations of cells, and a "copy" of each subpopulation
located throughout striate cortex to ensure that every property can be

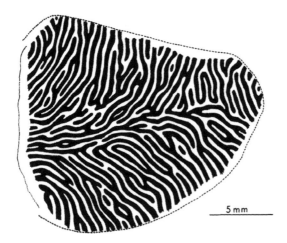

Figure 4.13
How information from the two eyes is combined in right occipital lobe of monkey visual cortex. Looking down on the surface of the cortex, input from the left eye is represented by black stripes, and input from the right eye by white stripes. The right-hand side represents the fovea. Obtained by injecting radioactive amino acid into one eye, which is then transported along the visual pathway to eye-specific cells in striate cortex. Redrawn courtesy of the Nobel Foundation from Hubel 1981.

detected in every part of striate cortex, and therefore in every part of the retinal image.

Working with monkeys, Hubel and Wiesel have shown that, if one eye is kept closed and the other eye is exposed to black and white vertical gratings, the resultant pattern of activity in striate cortex looks nothing like the vertical stripes we might have expected. The cells sensitive to the grating size and orientation used have a high output, which forces them to absorb a relatively large amount of glucose circulating in the bloodstream. When this glucose is tagged with radioactive carbon atoms, the most active cells become most radioactive. And when the visual cortex is then sliced parallel to its surface and laid on a photographic plate for a few days, the locations of radioactive regions in striate cortex become visible as dark blobs (in the negative), as shown in the *autora-diograph* of figure 4.15a. Thus the brain's representation of the retinal image needn't look anything like that image. More generally, there's no reason to suppose that the brain's representation of anything should resemble that thing, any more than the word *sheep* should resemble a woolly mammal.

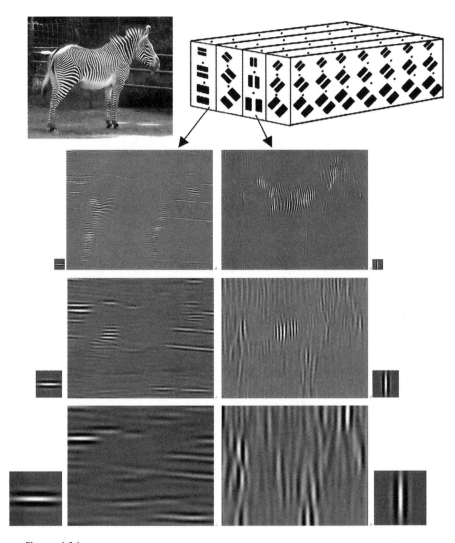

Figure 4.14

Hypothetical hypercolumns. Each small patch, or hyperfield, of the image (top left) is processed by a single hypercolumn (top right). Each hypercolumn includes simple cells with receptive fields with different sizes and orientations. Here, the outputs of three receptive field sizes, and two orientations (vertical and horizontal) are shown. The gray level at each point in each output image indicates the response of a simple cell with the receptive field shown at the lower corner of each image. Receptive fields of increasing size have been drawn in different cortical layers for display purposes only.

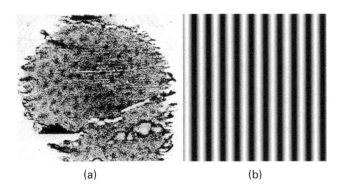

(a)   (b)

Figure 4.15
Activity in primary visual cortex (a) of a monkey induced by vertical grating (b) shown to one eye. The dark blobs therefore correspond to the intersection of two types of cells, those within orientation columns that respond to vertical lines, and those within ocularity stripes that belong only to the stimulated eye. The view shown corresponds to a horizontal slice parallel to the surface of the cortex. Reproduced with permission from Hubel & Wiesel 1979.

The Packing Problem

If all the information implicit in a retinal image is represented in the outputs of a million ganglion cells and if the cells of the visual cortex cannot add *new* information about the retinal image (and information theory assures us they cannot), then why are there 10 billion cells in the primary visual (striate) cortex?

The simple answer is that the information we need in order to see is only implicit in the information the cortex receives from the ganglion cells. Indeed, we have already seen how the outputs of a million ganglion cells are a compressed version of an image consisting of about 126 million photoreceptor outputs. So, in a sense, striate cortex provides a reexpansion of those outputs, except that it expands them well beyond the original 126 million photoreceptor outputs because it extracts features that are only implicit in the original retinal image (figure 4.16, plate 8). In other words, the task of the visual cortex is not to add information (which it cannot do), but to make explicit that which is merely implicit, as in figure 4.17 (e.g., to signal the presence of a long luminance edge from a line of adjacent ganglion cells). In a sense, when applied to complex visual entities, making the merely implicit explicit may be the principal task of the entire visual system.

One side-effect of making implicit image properties explicit is that all the newly extracted explicit data has to be represented somewhere, and

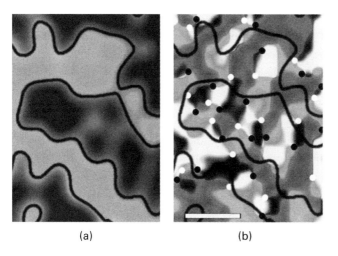

(a)   (b)

Figure 4.16 (plate 8)
Striate cortex as a polymap of different parameters. (a) Human ocularity map. (b) Color-coded orientation map. Both maps cover the same region of human striate cortex, and the black curves in (b) indicate the borders of the ocularity stripes also shown in (a), where dots indicate pinwheels. Obtained using functional magnetic resonance imaging (fMRI). Reproduced with permission from Yacoub, Harel, & Ugurbil 2008, copyright © 2008 National Academy of Sciences, USA.

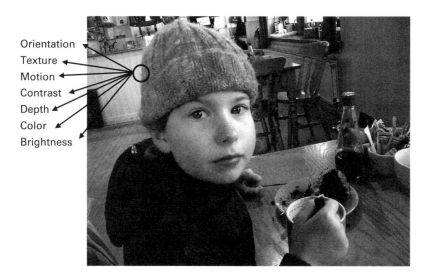

Figure 4.17
The need to make implicit features explicit in every point in the retinal image may explain the massive increase in neurons in primary visual cortex compared to the number of neurons sending information from the retina.

the result is the many maps observed in striate cortex. Given that all of these maps are overlaid within striate cortex, you might well ask, how do they all fit in? The answer to this question has two parts.

The first part is that they don't fit very well, which is why we witness the appearance of orientation singularities, described above. Hubel and Wiesel recognized that the brain is attempting to squeeze as many parameters as possible into the striate cortex. However, such an exercise is doomed to failure because it's mathematically impossible without creating singularities of one type or another (Pierce 1980, pp. 17, 179). Indeed, Hubel and Wiesel (1979) speculated that "perhaps the most plausible notion is that the column systems are a solution to the problem of portraying more than two dimensions in a two-dimensional surface."

The second part of the answer is that cells in different layers tend to represent different types of quantities. For example, simple cells tend to be in layer 4, whereas complex cells tend to reside in other layers. However, if the brain is able to detect every possible line orientation, every possible line direction and speed, and every possible line width (with both negative and positive contrasts) in every possible color, when presented to either eye, then it must have a cell capable of representing these properties at every possible location in the primary visual cortex. For obvious reasons, this is referred to as the "packing problem."

Given that each parameter is not stored in a separate layer within striate cortex, some savings can be obtained by an efficient meshing together of the different maps shown in figure 4.16 (plate 8). For example, the preferred orientation of cells varies smoothly from place to place across the striate cortex, but these smooth changes surround particular points, known as "orientation singularities" or "pinwheels," where there are sudden jumps in the preferred orientation of simple cells, as shown in figure 4.16. It turns out that these singularities in the orientation map are inevitable from a purely mathematical perspective. It therefore makes perfect sense for the cells at the center of each singularity to be used to represent some nonoriented parameter, which may explain why the majority of such cells seem to respond best to colors, as shown in figure 4.16.

The packing problem arises because the brain tries to assign several labels to every point in the image. For example, the edge of the hat in figure 4.17 has a particular color, texture, motion direction and speed, brightness, size, and orientation. Thus, even though each pixel in the image is defined by a single number (or three numbers for color images), once these more perceptually salient parameters have been made explicit, each pixel requires at least six numbers, each of which specifies the value of a different physical parameter. So, what began life as a two-dimensional retinal image, with one gray-level number per photoreceptor, is represented in striate cortex by at least six numbers per photoreceptor (assuming that the brain assigns a set of labels to every point or photoreceptor in the image).

To appreciate the fundamental nature of this problem, let's consider how the packing problem might be solved if the brain represented just line orientation at every point in the image. In this case, if different line orientations were represented at different layers within striate cortex, then the experiment described above using black and white stripes would yield activity in a single layer across all columns within striate cortex. In essence, retinal position would remain implicit and would be represented by position in striate cortex, whereas orientation would be represented by the activity of simple cells. Thus, by making use of the third dimension (i.e., cortical depth), the three parameters implicit in the retinal image (horizontal position, vertical position, and line orientation) could be adequately represented in striate cortex. However, we assumed the brain represented just one additional parameter, such as motion direction, we would find that the three-dimensional visual cortex had effectively run out of dimensions. If the universe had four spatial dimensions, instead of three, then this additional parameter would cause no problem. But even a four-dimensional cortex would encounter problems if it attempted to represent five parameters. Thus the packing problem arises not from the lack of dimensions in this particular universe but from the manifold richness of the representations constructed by the human brain. (If you need a quick review of one-, two-, and three-dimensional space, skip ahead to "Space, the First Frontier" in chapter 5).

The packing problem implies that the two-dimensional image in figure 4.17 requires a separate population of cells for every conceivable property or parameter (e.g., color, orientation) at every position in the image. If we assume that each image point has six parameters that the brain encodes, then it's as if every image really has a separate dimension for each parameter. Thus the two-dimensional image is really just a compact version of an eight-dimensional space (two dimensions for the image, and one for each of the six parameters). Two of the parameters can remain implicit because they are identified by their location within the retinotopic map in the primary visual cortex. But once the other, say, six parameters have been extracted within striate cortex, there is no room left to extract other, more perceptually salient parameters, like motion in depth, or faces.

Unless, that is, the brain treats other bits of cortex as spare representational space for these higher-order parameters.

Secondary Visual Cortex

The secondary visual cortex (V2) envelopes the striate cortex (V1). In area V2, we witness the start of a division of labor which becomes more marked as we progress through the visual system. Information in V2 is organized into parallel stripes. Staining for an enzyme called "cytochrome oxidase" reveals dark thick and thin stripes, separated by stripes that are pale because they contain relatively little cytochrome oxidase (these pale stripes are also called "interstripes"). These three types of stripes received projections from specific parts of V1, as shown in figure 4.7.

The thin stripes receive their inputs from color *blobs* in striate cortex. As you might predict from the response characteristics of cells in color blobs, cells in thin stripes are sensitive to color or brightness, but not to orientation. The thick stripes receive their inputs from layer 4B of striate cortex, which is part of the magno (M) pathway. Consequently, cells in the thick stripes respond to specific orientations, but not to color. A key property of these cells is that they are binocular. They are driven by inputs from both eyes and respond best when a line projects to a slightly different position on each retina. This difference or disparity in the retinal positions of lines suggests that these cells represent binocular disparity. The pale interstripes of V2 receive their inputs from the complex and hypercomplex cells in striate cortex. Because these cells receive their inputs from the parvocellular layers of the LGN, they respond best to oriented lines. Despite this division of labor within V2, adjacent stripes respond to the same region of retina, ensuring that the retinotopic map found in striate cortex is approximately preserved in V2.

Color Cortex

The thin stripes and interstripes of V2, both of which belong to the parvocellular (P) stream, project to the "color area" V4. The quotation marks are used to indicate that cells in V4 respond not only to color but also to simple shapes and objects. This means that V4 has to find a way to squeeze retinal location, color, and shape parameters into a two-dimensional space. As we shall see in figure 4.19, V4 seems not to have an accurate retinotopic map, probably because its primary concern is color and shape, rather than retinal location. Thus, in V4, we may be witnessing the decline of retinal location as the dominant organizing principle, and the rise of feature-based cortical maps, which use color or shape as their dominant organizing principle.

The dominant organizing principle for a given cortical map is called its *primary index*. For example, within striate cortex, the primary index is spatial (because the structure of this map is dominated by retinal position), whereas its secondary indices include color and orientation.

Motion Cortex

The thick stripes of V2, which belong to the magnocellular (M) stream, project to the "motion area" V5. Again, the quotation marks are used to indicate that cells in V5 not only respond to motion; they also respond to other parameters, especially stereo disparity, as shown in figure 4.18 (plate 9); for an account of stereo disparity, skip ahead to "Stereo Vision" in chapter 5).Thus, just as each cell in striate cortex has a preferred orientation, so each cell in V5 has a particular range of preferred speeds, directions, and disparity values.

In one of the few experiments to show that cells responding to a specific visual parameter affect the perception of that parameter, C. Daniel Salzman

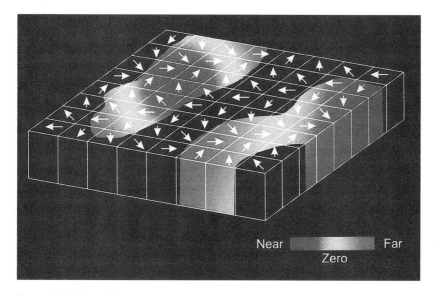

Figure 4.18 (plate 9)
Area MT (V5) codes for motion and stereo disparity. Schematic diagram in which arrows show the preferred direction and color shows the stereo disparity of cells. The terms "near" and "far" refer to the amount of stereo disparity. Reproduced with permission from DeAngelis & Newsome 1999.

and colleagues (1992) observed that the cells in V5 seem to mediate decisions regarding perceived motion. They trained monkeys to indicate whether dots on a screen were moving up or down on a screen. From previous results, Salzman knew that cells in area V5 identified as having, say, an upward preferred direction, would increase their outputs when the dots moved upward. But when a small electrical current was injected into these cells while the monkey was making a decision about the direction of the dots, the monkey's responses shifted exactly as if *extra* dots with upward motion had been added to the screen. In other words, this *microstimulation* of cells with a preferred upward direction acted as a proxy for actual motion. Gregory DeAngelis, Bruce Cumming, and William Newsome (2000) performed a similar experiment on monkeys using judgments based on stereo depth, with similar results. These elegant experiments provide evidence that V5 is not just an idle bystander, but seems to be *causally involved* in the perception of motion and stereo. This may count as the ultimate (if primitive) virtual reality. Just as V4 has reduced *retinotopy* (point-for-point mapping of cortical to retinal neurons), so the relative lack of retinotopy in V5 may exemplify how the purely spatial primary index apparent in V1 (striate cortex) and V2 may be replaced by the non-spatial primary index of motion in V5.

Losing Retinotopy

Although there's little doubt that the striate cortex provides a reasonably accurate map of the retinal image, other visual areas seem to supplant this retinotopy with some other property. Evidence for the loss of retinotopy can be obtained by making use of the following logic: given a perfect retinotopic map, if a straight line is drawn across striate cortex then it should pass through a sequence of neurons with a corresponding sequence of receptive fields that lie on a straight line *on the retina*. Using this logic, Semir Zeki (1993) drove a microelectrode across and just beneath the surface of striate cortex in a monkey. Then, at regular intervals, he stopped with the electrode inside a single neuron. By probing the retina (e.g., using a spot of light) he then found which part of the retina could induce activity in this neuron, and therefore how each electrode location in the cortex mapped to a corresponding retinal location. For striate cortex, he found that the straight-line penetration across the cortex yielded a corresponding line that was almost straight on the retina, as shown in figure 4.19.

Zeki then repeated this process with straight-line penetrations across visual regions V2, V4, and V5. As can be seen from figure 4.19, the corresponding paths across the retina became more chaotic as Zeki tested

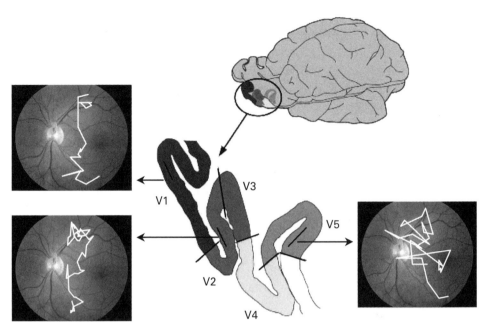

Figure 4.19
Losing retinotopy. Straight-line electrode track parallel to the surface of the striate cortex (area V1), shown as a straight line across V1, maps to a corresponding path on the retina, shown in white here. The retinal path for a straight-line electrode track across cortical regions V2 and V5 maps to a corresponding path on the retina. Only the straight-line electrode track across V1 yields a fairly straight path across the retina. These paths are not drawn to scale. Modified with permission from Zeki 1993.

regions "farther" from striate cortex. One explanation for this loss of retinotopy is that the primary and secondary indexes gradually swap places as we move away from the striate cortex. That is, the striate cortex strives hard to retain information regarding where on the retina events occur, as evidenced by its spatial primary index. In contrast, an area such as V5 (which maintains some degree of retinotopy) is probably more concerned with motion across the retina and less concerned with exactly where this motion occurs. In other words, as we move away from the striate cortex, a new agenda gradually supplants the simplistic low-level description offered by the striate cortex.

Although this represents a speculative account, it has some merit. The deeper question is, if nonstriate areas don't have retinal location as their primary index, what *is* their primary index?

Inferotemporal Cortex

The stunning response characteristics of cells in inferotemporal cortex speak for themselves, as they do in figures 4.20 and 4.21 (plates 10 and 11). In figure 4.20, each point in a small region of inferotemporal cortex seems to represent a different view of a face. But perhaps the most surprising finding is that nearby cells respond to *similar* views of the face. In other words, it's as if the primary index of inferotemporal cortex is not retinal location at all but a highly abstract parameter, namely, viewpoint.

What if different cells responded to different views of your grandmother, and what if the outputs of all these cells converged on a single cell? Surely, this cell would respond to any view of your grandmother and to no other individuals. Such a cell has long been the topic of debate within the vision community, and is known as the "grandmother cell," a concept

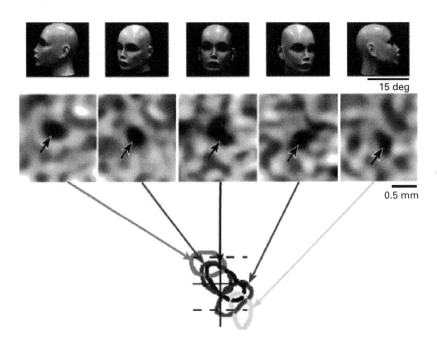

Figure 4.20 (plate 10)
Face-view cells in inferotemporal cortex. The view shown at the top evokes activity in cortex (middle row) at a location shown by the dark spot. The cortical locations of these spots have been overlaid at the bottom to shown how similar views evoke activity in adjacent cortical regions. This suggests that nearby cortical locations represent similar face views. Reproduced with permission from Tanaka 2004; Wang, Tanaka, & Tanifuji 1996.

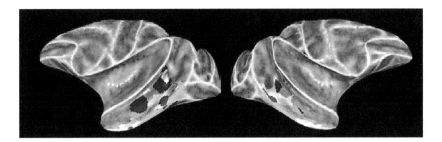

Figure 4.21 (plate 11)
Inflated views of the monkey brain showing regions of inferotemporal cortex selective for faces (red), body parts (yellow), objects (green), and places (blue). Reproduced with permission from Bell et al. 2009.

introduced by Jerome Lettvin around 1969. As an increasing number of cells were discovered that responded to increasingly abstract visual features, the idea of a grandmother cell seemed to be logically inevitable. Indeed, if the visual system consisted of a hierarchy of cells that responded to increasingly abstract parameters then neurons like the grandmother cell would stand at the top of that hierarchy. However, it's worth noting that the existence of such a cell creates as many problems as it appears to solve (for example, what if the cell died?).

Recently, Rodrigo Quian Quiroga and colleagues (2005) seem to have discovered a candidate for a neuron that behaves like a grandmother cell. During surgery for epilepsy, they monitored the output of cells in a patient's inferotemporal cortex while the patient was shown images of various faces. One cell seemed to respond only to images of Jennifer Aniston from the TV series *Friends*. However, it is far from clear what role, if any, such a cell has to play in the process of perception. Interestingly, nearby cells did not seem to respond to different views of Aniston, but they did respond to other characters in *Friends*. As will be described in chapter 9, this suggests that nearby cells may represent a set of parameters that occur nearby in time, where "parameter" here refers to the identity of a person, a very high order parameter indeed.

The interesting implication of this finding is that the view-selective cortical cells describe above may also be organized according to temporal context. Nearby cells represent similar views. But notice that views represented by cells that are next to one another on the cortex are usually experienced as being near to one another in time. In other words, the *temporal proximity* of views experienced in everyday life may be reflected in the physical proximity of the cortical cells that represent those views.

One possible objection to this line of reasoning is that the temporal sequence of different views of a turning head occurs over seconds, whereas the appearance of Aniston followed by her costars occurs over minutes. However, it remains an intriguing possibility that the high-order "feature maps" observed in inferotemporal cortex are supported by the temporal proximity of visual inputs rather than by their similarity in terms of some high-order parameter, such as viewpoint or even person identity. And it's worth noting that this approach has received support from computational models of learning in cortex (see chapter 6).

Other high-order features that seem to be represented in inferotemporal cortex include hands, faces, walking humans, and objects, with different types of objects represented in different regions of inferotemporal cortex. That said, there does seem to be a coherent map of related objects within each small region. As with other extrastriate areas, the retinotopy of the map in inferotemporal cortex seems to be quite eroded, although, given the difficulty of determining what each cell represents, making precise feature maps of large regions of inferotemporal cortex is still very much a "work in progress."

A Mill and a Grand Book

The research program that followed Hubel and Wiesel's discoveries has been extraordinarily successful. However, this success has been tempered by the growing realization that describing how the components of a system work is not the same as understanding exactly how the system as a whole works. This realization was foreshadowed by the German philosopher and co-inventor with Isaac Newton of calculus, Gottfried Leibniz (1646–1716):

Let us pretend that there was a machine, which was constructed in such a way as to give rise to thinking, sensing, and having perceptions. You could imagine it expanded in size . . . , so that you could go inside it, like going into a mill. On this assumption, your tour inside it would show you the working parts pushing each other, but never anything which would explain a perception. (Leibniz 1714; in Rescher 1991)

If we could only dig deeper into the secrets of brain, would we then understand how vision works? There are at least two types of answer to this question, a short one and a long one. The short answer is implicit in the words of one of the first scientists:

Philosophy is written in this grand book—the universe—which stands continuously open to our gaze. But the book cannot be understood unless one first learns to comprehend the language and interpret the characters in which it is written. It is written in the language of mathematics ... without which it is humanly impossible to understand a single word of it; without these one is wandering about in a dark labyrinth. (Galileo Galilei [1564–1642], *The Assayer* in Machamer 1998, 64–65).

Or, to put it in modern terms, if we think we understand any system then we should be able to devise a precise mathematical model of it. Given such a mathematical model, we should be able to build a model of the system that, when given inputs, yields outputs matching those of the system under consideration. This model could be a physical model (e.g., an android) or a computer emulation of a physical process (e.g., weather systems).

The long answer would involve an analysis of what it means to understand anything, beyond a theory expressed only in words. The problem is that such a purely linguistic account can be a slippery creature, and in the absence of a mathematical formulation of a given theory, we are left with Galileo's words for guidance.

With regard to vision, the foremost protagonist of the Galilean approach was David Marr. Marr proposed that vision requires a rigorous analysis which takes account of findings from physiology, physics, and psychophysics, but which ultimately must be capable of solving the fundamental problems that confront any visual system.

5 Depth: The Rogue Dimension

Every body in light and shade fills the surrounding air with infinite images of itself.
—Leonardo da Vinci (1452–1519), Notebooks

Impressions

It is no distance from the image of an upheld coin to the halo of moonshine beyond. No distance across the retina. Less than a small step for a man, but a quarter of a million miles, and a giant leap for the brain to know that distances exist beyond the confines of the retinal image, and out, into space.

Seeing is not a passive process. It requires work. Not just mental work measured in who-knows-what units, but physical work required to generate and sustain action potentials; work that is measured in joules or calories. More importantly, seeing requires computational work, which also translates into calories. The amount of computational and therefore physical work required to sustain the brain is so enormous that it has been suggested that the major limiting factor with regard to brain function is not size or weight but the energy required to keep it running.

In essence, brain tissue is probably the most energetically expensive tissue in the animal kingdom, and this has two main consequences. First, having a bigger brain requires a bigger intake of food. In other words, each extra gram of brain costs extra energy, and this cost must be balanced by the Darwinian fitness benefits it brings: it must earn its way. Second, the large energy requirements of neuronal action potentials mean that brain cells should be active as little as possible; that is, the number of action potentials per neuron should be kept to an absolute minimum.

And what does all this work achieve? From an evolutionary perspective, it achieves an extra toehold on Darwin's ever-changing cliff face of Mount Fitness. But the brain's goal of seeing is achieved by satisfying a plethora of computational sub-goals, which consist in transforming retinal images into information about the physical world. More precisely, it consists in making explicit all of the perceptually salient information that is merely implicit in the stream of images that pass across the retinas. In essence, it consists in creating a particular representation of the visual world inside our heads, although it is unlikely that this representation is anything like the pictorial nature of the retinal image. In this chapter, we explore the perceptual cues that contribute to this representation of the visual world.

Space, the First Frontier

One of the central problems of vision is that the world we see is full of depth, but the retinal image is flat. It is as if the dimension of depth gets squeezed out just as the light from the three-dimensional world hits the retina. Somehow, that missing dimension has to be reconstituted from the fragments of clues that the two-dimensional retinal image retains about the 3-D world from which it originated.

Before explaining why this part of vision is so very hard, we should first define exactly what is meant by a two- and a three-dimensional space. To do this, let's begin with a zero-dimensional space, a point. Put an infinite set of points in a row, and you have a one-dimensional space, a line. The position of a point on a line can be specified with a single number. For example, the position of a small object, like a spider, on the line running along the edge of a freeway as its distance from the start of the freeway—a single number. If you know that number then you know where the spider is.

A two-dimensional space is a flat plane, like a football field or a door. The position of a point in a 2-D space can be specified with two numbers. For example, if we define the lower hinge corner of a door as the origin then we can give the position of a spider on the door as its distance from the origin along the horizontal or x-axis and along the vertical or y-axis. If you know those two numbers or two-dimensional *coordinates* then you know where the spider is located on the door.

A three-dimensional space is a volume, like the room in figure 5.1. The position of a point in a 3-D space can be specified with three numbers. First, we define the origin to be at one corner on the floor. Now, the position of any point (or spider) is given by its distance from the origin above the floor—height—along the vertical axis (the Y-axis), distance along one wall as one horizontal axis (the X-axis), and distance along another wall—depth—as the other horizontal axis (the Z-axis). If you know those three numbers or three-dimensional coordinates then you know where the spider is located in the room.

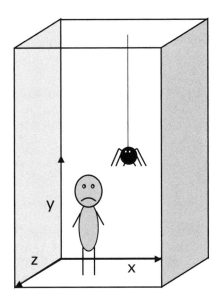

Figure 5.1
A room as three-dimensional space. The *X*-axis defines position from left to right, the *Y*-axis from bottom to top, and the *Z*-axis from back to front (depth). A spider requires three numbers, the distance from the origin along the *X*-, *Y*-, and *Z*-axes to specify its position in the room (e.g., [*X, Y, Z*] = [3, 2, 1]). By definition, the origin is located at [0, 0, 0].

Painting Pictures on the Retina

When light falls out of the three-dimensional world and onto your retina, it paints a picture, but it's a two-dimensional picture. And as everyone knows, three into two won't go. What's true for whole numbers (integers) turns out to be true for dimensions as well.

It is not possible, even in principle, to squeeze all the points in a three-dimensional space into a two-dimensional space without introducing severe distortions in the form of breaks or *discontinuities* (Pierce, 1980). For example, adjacent points on the surface of a cube, say, 3 meters on a side, always project to adjacent points in an image of that cube. But a pair of points in the image can be derived from two points separated by several miles in the world, because one of the image points could be at the edge of the cube and the other one could be on a cloud behind the cube. So whereas adjacent points in the 3-D world always yield adjacent points in the 2-D image, adjacent points in the 2-D image could come from points separated by miles in the 3-D world. In other words, there's a *continuous* mapping from the world to the image, but a *discontinuous* mapping from the image to the world.

A less extreme, but more common, consequence of this discontinuous mapping is that adjacent points with different depths on the surface of an object end up as adjacent points in the retinal image. But these points from different depths do not carry depth labels; they are just points like any other points in the image. The depth information is lost or at least mixed in with other types of information regarding texture, color, and line orientation. Much, perhaps most, of vision is concerned with reconstituting this missing dimension of depth by adding water to each desiccated two-dimensional image to retrieve the three-dimensional information hiding within it.

Pictorial Cues to Distance

When you look at a scene like figure 5.2 or figure 5.3, you can easily see which objects are more distant and which are closer to the camera. Precisely how you know which objects are farther away depends on a few obvious cues, like size, as well as some more subtle ones, like the height

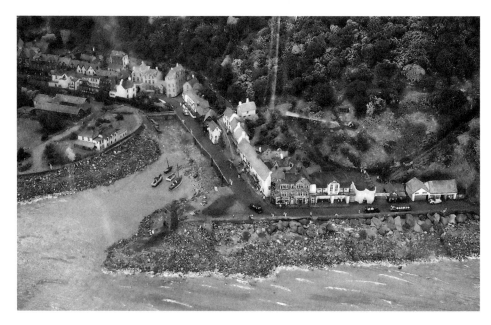

Figure 5.2
Pictorial cues give information about *relative* depth and size, which makes it hard to judge the absolute size of objects in this model of the village of Lynmouth, England.

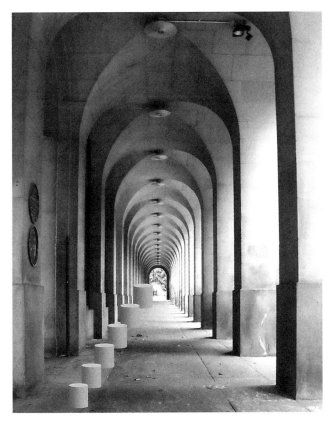

Figure 5.3
Size invariance. The columns on the left-hand side have been added to the original picture. Every column is the same size on the page, and the distance between adjacent columns is the same on the page.

of an object in an image. The cues that provide information about depth in such scenes are called "pictorial cues."

Let's begin with the obvious cues. Clearly, if one object is in front of another then your view of that object is obscured or *occluded*, so that occlusion tells you about the relative depth of objects, as in figure 5.3. The drum-shaped objects in figure 5.3 appear to get larger as they recede into the distance. However, these drums have been added to the photograph and are the *same* size on the page. Because the receding arches give the impression that some drums are farther away, you perceive them as being *bigger* in the *world*.

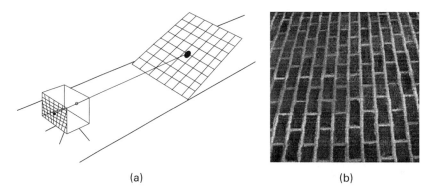

(a)   (b)

Figure 5.4

Geometric origin of the texture gradient. (a) Squares on more distant regions of a plane get squeezed into a small image region creating a high density of image texture (at the bottom of the inverted image). Because distance varies continuously, there is a continuous change in image texture density, and this texture gradient increases with increasingly slanted surfaces. From Frisby & Stone 2010. (b) Typical image of a slanted plane.

If you are looking at a scene that contains texture then the rate at which texture changes across the image tells you about the slant of surfaces in that scene. For example, because the wall in figure 5.4 has the same number of bricks or *texture elements* for each square meter of its surface, its *texture density* is uniform or *homogeneous*. But the texture density of its image *increases* with distance, and the resultant *texture gradient* tells us precisely how much the wall is slanted with respect to the camera. Indeed, because image texture density increases with the cube of depth (i.e., with Z^3), doubling the distance increases the image texture density eight-fold.

Thus knowing the texture density of different image regions tells us about the relative depth of the corresponding regions in the world. In practice, we need to measure the density in at least three image regions to estimate the orientation of a planar surface like a wall, but the principle for doing so remains the same: the image texture density varies predictably, in a systematic manner, and the nature of this systematic change across the image can be used to estimate surface orientation. These changes in texture density cannot be used to compute the *distance* to a point in the world (e.g., on a wall), they only tell us about *relative* distances. Other cues to depth in a scene, such as motion and stereo, aren't classed as pictorial cues because they do not provide depth information from a single static image. These nonpictorial cues will be explored next.

Motion: What is It Good For?

The frog does not seem to see or, at any rate, is not concerned with the detail of stationary parts of the world around him. He will starve to death surrounded by food if it is not moving.

—Jerome Lettvin and colleagues (1959)

Before considering *how* we might perceive motion, we should first explore *why* we need to perceive motion at all. The epigraph for this section exemplifies a common feature of vision: if an object doesn't move then we are often blind to its existence. The importance of motion is supported by the finding that even new-born infants are startled by a pattern of dots that expand out from the center, suggesting that they recognize such a looming pattern as implying a surface is moving rapidly toward them, as in figure 5.5.

Now You See It . . .

Just as the visual system is excellent at seeing things at a specific range of sizes or spatial frequencies, so it also has a range of rates of change or *temporal frequencies* that it's especially good at seeing. The extent to which the visual system "likes" particular rates of change can be measured in the form of a flickering black and white disk, as shown in figure 5.6a. The flicker rate or temporal frequency is measured as the number of times the

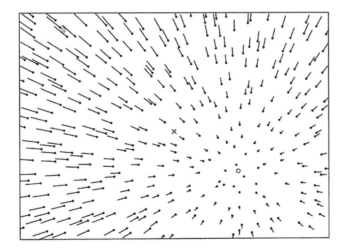

Figure 5.5

Pattern of optic flow resulting from motion, as if the observer is traveling into a tunnel. Reproduced with permission from Warren 2004.

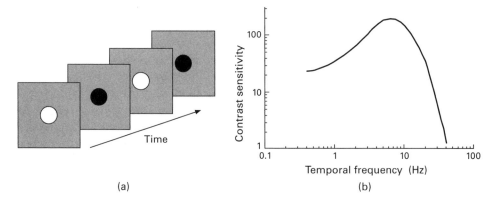

(a)   (b)

Figure 5.6
Temporal contrast sensitivity function. (a) Measuring performance at a single flicker
rate (temporal frequency), defined in changes from black to white per second or
hertz (Hz). From Frisby & Stone 2010. (b) Ability to detect flicker at different flicker
rates defines the temporal contrast sensitivity function. Note both axes are logarithmic. Reproduced with permission from de Lange 1958.

disk executes one full *cycle* from black to white and back to black each
second. If this occurs, say, 10 times a second then the temporal frequency
is 10 hertz (Hz).

We obtain the visual system's *sensitivity* to a particular temporal frequency by reducing the contrast of the disks until no flicker is perceived.
The smallest perceivable contrast at each flicker rate is the *contrast threshold*
for that particular flicker rate, and the system's sensitivity to it (plotted in
figure 5.6b) is the *reciprocal* of that threshold or 1/(contrast threshold).

The graph in figure 5.6b shows that we have the highest temporal resolution for changes that happen about 10 times per second, or 10 Hz. It
also shows that we're almost blind to changes above about 30 Hz, which
is why we see the images in a movie, projected at a 24 frames per second,
as continuous motion, rather than as the sequence of static images they
really are.

Staying Upright

Seeing motion is not only useful for knowing if things in the world are
moving; it also helps us know if *we* are moving. One demonstration of the
importance of motion detection involves a toddler and a cruel deception,
as shown in figure 5.7. A toddler is placed in the middle of a room in which
the walls and ceiling form a solid suspended a few inches above the floor.
While the toddler is wondering what's going on, the suspended walls are

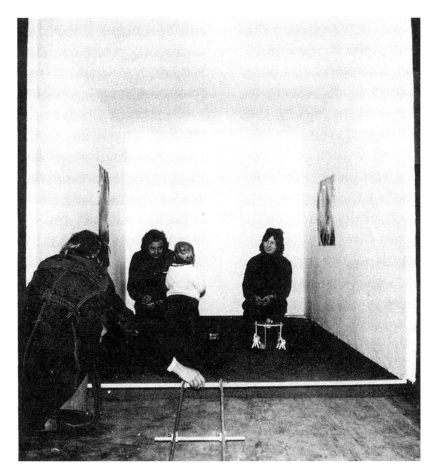

Figure 5.7
How to make a toddler fall over. While the toddler is distracted by two adults, the adult in the foreground makes the ceiling and walls of the "room" sway back and forth. Reproduced with permission from Lee & Aronson 1974.

gently pushed back and forth. As they move, so does the toddler. The walls sway, the toddler sways. When the walls are pushed harder, the toddler sways even more and then falls over. Without being aware of it, the toddler uses the walls as visual reference points. If all of the walls appear to move in one direction, say northward, then his brain infers that this must be because his body is leaning southward, and his brain tries to compensate for this by leaning his body northward. However, as he was initially perfectly vertical, this compensatory lean takes him away from vertical, until, much to his surprise, he becomes horizontal.

Motion Parallax and Optic Flow

If you move your head from side to side while looking at a point on the horizon then objects close to you appear to move in the opposite direction to your head's motion (this also works if you look at the farthest point in a room). More importantly, the *amount* of apparent motion of objects decreases with distance, until finally, when objects are at the same distance as the point you are looking at, they do not appear to move at all. This is an example of *motion parallax*, and its effects tell you about the relative distances of objects in the world. More formally, motion parallax is caused by the differential speed with which stationary objects move across the retinal image, a speed which depends on their distances from a moving observer looking at a single point (called the "fixation point") in the world (figure 5.8).

Most of us can see depth because we have two views of the world, one from each eye, which we can use to estimate relative depth using *stereopsis* (see "Stereo Vision" below). If we had only one of these two views then we would be forced to fall back on other cues to depth, like motion parallax. Indeed, the utility of motion parallax as a cue to depth may well

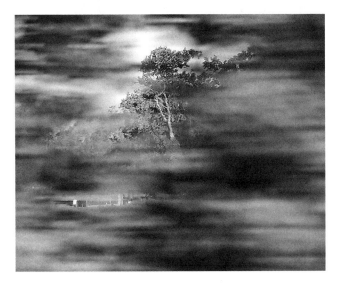

Figure 5.8
Extreme example of motion parallax. This picture was taken from a moving train. The bushes in the foreground are blurred by their rapid motion across the image, whereas the trees in the background remain relatively sharp. Reproduced with permission.

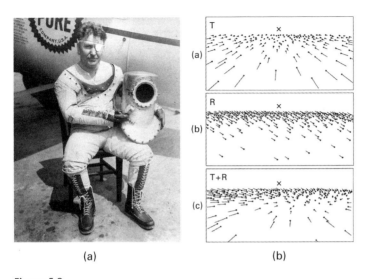

(a)   (b)

Figure 5.9
(a) Wiley Post, shown here wearing an early high-altitude pressure suit, made the
first solo flight around the world in less than eight days during 1933, despite having
only one eye. (b) When a pilot lands a plane, the pattern of optic flow on the retina
informs the pilot's brain about the relative depths of different points in a scene.
Reproduced with permission from Warren 2004.

explain how Wiley Post (figure 5.9) managed to make the first solo flight
around the world in 1933, even though he had only one eye.

Precisely how Wiley Post, or any pilot, achieves a smooth landing can
be understood in terms of insect flight. When an insect flies toward a
particular point, the visual world appears to flow around the insect, with
nearby points having greater speed across the eye's images than distant
points. This *optic flow field* has zero speed only at the point to which the
insect is heading, and it is therefore called the "focus of expansion." For a
pilot, the early stages of a smooth landing can therefore be achieved by
ensuring that the flight path is continually adjusted so that the far end of
the runway is kept in the center of the focus of expansion. Obviously, the
later stages of a landing require adjustments to ensure that the plane's nose
does not hit the runway.

Bees famously communicate the location of a food source by means of
a waggle dance, as shown in figure 5.10. The waggle dance consists of
repeated waggles along a particular direction, usually within the nest. The
direction of a bee's waggle specifies the direction relative to the sun,
whereas the duration of the dance within each repeat of the dance specifies

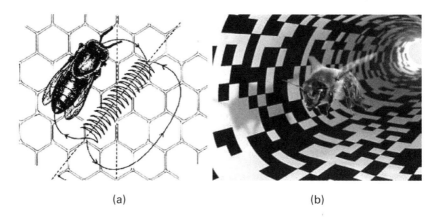

(a)   (b)

Figure 5.10
Bees use optic flow to measure distance. (a) The waggle dance of the bee tells other bees where to find food. The direction of the food is indicated by the direction of the dance, whereas the distance to the food is related to the duration of the dance along the chosen direction. (b) Because this "distance" seems to be measured in terms of the amount of optic flow encountered by the dancing bee on her way to the food, placing a fine texture in a tunnel that leads to a food source makes the bee think she has traveled farther than she really has.

the distance to the food source. However, the relationship between the dance duration and the distance to the food source is quite subtle. It is communicated not in units of meters or inches, but by the amount of optical flow the bee encountered on her way to the food source (worker bees are sterile females).

In an ingeneous experiment, Harald Esch, Shaowu Zhang, Mandyan Srinivasan, and Juergen Tautz (2001) placed a tunnel between a bee hive and a food source, so that bees had to fly through this tunnel to collect food. If the tunnel is painted with a fine texture, then the bee is fooled into "thinking" she has traveled a long way, as indicated by the longer duration of her waggle dance. Conversely, if the tunnel contains a coarse texture, then the bee seems to "think" she has traveled a short distance, because her waggle dance has a shorter duration. In other words, the bee mistakes distance for the amount of optic flow experienced during a flight to a food source.

A similar trick is used to slow drivers down when approaching junctions or intersections. Making the gaps between painted lines across the road smaller fools the driver into thinking the car is moving faster than it really is. So the visual cues that govern how far bees think they've traveled also

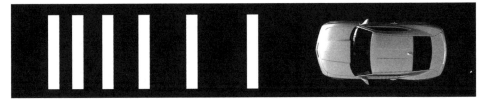

Figure 5.11
Optic flow. The shrinking spaces between stripes on the road gives the illusion of increasing speed for a car driving from right to left in the picture, and may encourage drivers to slow down when approaching junctions.

govern how fast we think we're moving. Bees and humans confront the same problems, so it is no surprise that they use the same visual cues to judge distances, and that they are fooled by the same visual tricks, as in figure 5.11.

The optics of vision dictate that the retinal speed s of an object at an optic angle θ (theta) from the insect's heading direction (i.e., from the focus of expansion) is determined by the insect's speed v, and the object's distance d. For objects that are almost straight ahead, a "small angle" approximation yields $d \approx v\theta/s$ (where the symbol $\approx$ means "approximately equal").

This equation holds true not only for insects in flight but also for pilots trying to land a plane and for you as you walk along while keeping your eyes fixed on a specific point in a scene, which is the center of your focus of expansion. In essence, it means that, if you know the speed at which an object is crossing your retinal image, the angle between the object and your focus of expansion, and your own speed then your brain can, in principle, work out the *exact* distance to that object.

Of course, you do not have to be flying an airplane or walking along in order to estimate the distance to an object. Any motion will do, like moving your head from side to side, or back and forth. Side-to-side head motion or *peering* is used by locusts when estimating the distance needed to jump on to an object. This was demonstrated by Eric Sobel (1990), who artificially reduced the amount of motion the locust sees by moving the object from side-to-side in synchrony with the locust's head movements. When this is done, the locust jumps too far, as if it is fooled into thinking that the object is closer than it really is, confirming that locusts use motion parallax to judge distances (Sobel, 1990).

The equation given above specifies how any device that makes use of optic flow must operate at a computational level. In other words, any device that relies on optic flow is bound by the form of the equation given above, which has one more general lesson for us. Once we have formulated the problem of finding distances using this equation, we have crossed a threshold in terms of our understanding. Moreover, this threshold applies to almost any analysis that transforms our initial intuitions into an equation. To take a simple example, the arc of a cannon ball as it flies through the air is governed by an equation, even though the precise form of that equation does not matter for our purposes. The point is that once we have this equation, we can work out the trajectory of almost any object: a ball, a rock, or a rocket. And we can do this for any object on any planet; the Earth, Mars, or Jupiter. In other words, a precise mathematical formulation of a problem often yields a similarly precise mathematical solution that is essentially decoupled from the particulars of the original problem. We may begin by trying to work out how to hit our enemy with a cannon ball when fired from an iron cannon, but if we are thorough then our solution tells us how to fire a rocket at the moon, and the trajectory of any object on any planet when fired from anything that can launch an object upward. This is the lesson that a computational analysis has to offer: the ability to decouple the particular details of one instance of a problem from the general principles that underpin its solution.

The Motion Aftereffect

Next time you are in a train station, wait for a train to pull in on the opposite track. As it pulls away, keep your eyes fixed on a single point above the train, so that the image of the departing train streaks across your retinas. Whatever comes into view after the last carriage has left appears to move in the *opposite* direction to that of the departed train. This is the *motion aftereffect*, which can also be observed with waterfalls and with roads viewed from a moving car.

Aristotle (ca. 330 BC) was the first to accurately describe the motion aftereffect, which was then forgotten until the nineteenth century. It was later rediscovered several times, notably by Jan Evangelista Purkinje (1825): "One time I observed a cavalry parade for more than an hour, and then when the parade had passed, the houses directly opposite appeared to me to move in the reversed direction to the parade." A few years later, Robert Addams (1834) described a similar effect after gazing for some time at the Fall of Foyers waterfall in Scotland, and the effect thereafter became known as the "waterfall illusion."

A Neuronal Model of the Motion Aftereffect

Both Sigmund Exner (1894) and Adolf Wohlgemuth (1911) devised models not much different from the model in figure 5.12. The basic idea is that

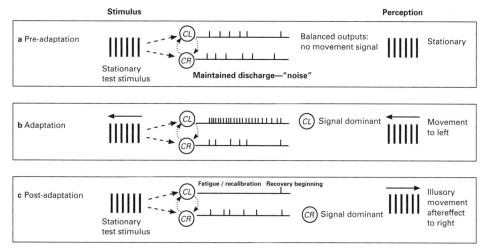

Figure 5.12
Explanation of the motion aftereffect described by Exner (1894) in terms of modern knowledge about neurons sensitive to motion. From Frisby & Stone 2010.

motion perception along a particular axis relies on a comparison between an *opposing pair* of motion detecting neurons. For example, motion along a horizontal axis could be detected using a pair of cells, CL with a firing rate r_L, which detects motion to the left, and CR with a firing rate r_R, which detects motion to the right. If the stimulus of vertical bar is stationary then both cells have a baseline firing rate, so that $r_L \approx r_R$. Thus the perceived motion in this *pre-adaptation* period is zero.

During an *adaptation* period, the stimulus moves leftward, causing CL's firing rate to increase, so that r_L is greater than r_R (i.e., $r_L > r_R$), and a leftward motion is perceived. However, when the motion stops, the cell CL is assumed to have become fatigued in some way, with the result that its output falls *below baseline* during a *post-adaptation* recovery period. In contrast, because the output r_R of CR remains at baseline, CR's output r_R is greater than CL's output r_L. If motion perception depends on a comparison between the *opponent pair* of cell outputs r_L and r_R then an illusory *rightward* motion should be perceived during this post-adaptation period during which $r_R > r_L$.

The general idea that motion perception relies on a comparison between opponent pairs of cells has received some experimental support (e.g., Carandini, Heeger, & Movshon 1997). On the other hand, the hypothesis that *fatigue* underlies the reduced output of a cell seems naive, if not downright suspect, in the context of modern computational theories of perception. Because the motion aftereffect can be apparent even 26 hours after a 15-minute adaptation period (Masland 1969), such a hypothesis would require cells to show signs of fatigue after a full day, which seems unlikely. Moreover, a post-adaptation period of complete darkness maintains the aftereffect long after it would normally have disappeared (an effect known as "storage"). The fatigue hypothesis would require that darkness somehow prevents recovery from neuronal fatigue. Again, this seems unlikely.

A more principled approach involves measuring the amount of *information* conveyed about motion. Surprisingly, experiments on single neurons in flies suggest that the reduced firing rate following adaptation to motion has the effect of *increasing* a neuron's total information about that motion (Brenner, Bialek, & de Ruyter van Steveninck, 2000). Thus, the observed changes in sensitivity of neurons to motion may be a side-effect of neurons attempting to convey as much information as possible in their outputs.

To return briefly to the topic of opponency, there's a striking similarity between a pair of cells being sensitive to motion in opposite directions and a pair of ganglion cells being sensitive to positive and negative contrasts (i.e., to opposite contrasts). Recall that opponent processing by retinal ganglion cells can yield neuronal outputs that collectively overcome the nonlinearities implicit in neurons, so that their outputs increase in direct proportion to contrast in the retinal image. Similarly, it seems plausible that the opponent processing suggested by the existence of the motion aftereffect yields neuronal outputs that reduce motion-related nonlinearities, allowing collective cell outputs to increase in direct proportion to motion on the retina (although it shoud be noted that there is, as yet, no evidence for this). We'll encounter similar types of opponency when we consider color perception.

Motion Blur

Motion blur is caused either by an object that's moving fast past a stationary eye (camera), as in figure 5.8, or by an eye (camera) that's moving fast past a stationary scene, as in figure 5.13. The result of motion blur is an image that looks out of focus, but this lack of focus occurs in just one orientation across the image, along the direction of motion, as shown in figure 5.8. The fact that motion blur and focus blur look similar provides a clue as to the origins of motion blur. To understand why this similarity exists, we first need to consider *focus blur*.

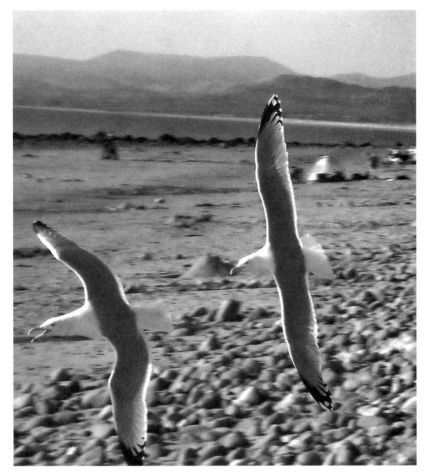

Figure 5.13
Motion blur. The blurred background is caused by the rapid motion of the camera
as it tracks the motion of the seagulls.

Focus blur is caused by each point in a scene being smeared out over
many photoreceptors, such that many scene points contribute to the input
to each photoreceptor, as in figure 5.14. Thus each photoreceptor input is
the average luminance of many points in a scene. Similarly, when a camera
is moving fast, the interval during which the camera shutter is open causes
each scene point to be smeared out along a line of photoreceptors *in the
direction of motion*; conversely, many scene points aligned along the direction of motion contribute to the input to each photoreceptor.

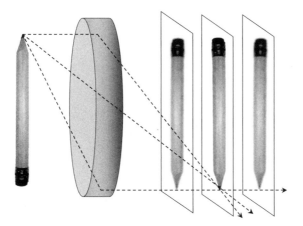

Figure 5.14
Focus blur. If an image plane is at the correct distance from the lens, each point in the scene projects to a single point in the image. But if it's at any other distance then the image is blurred because each point in the scene gets smeared out in all directions over a relatively large region in the image.

So why do we experience motion blur? Because each photoreceptor needs a small interval of time to build up its response to the light from the small patch of scene that happens to be hitting it. This interval effectively acts like a fixed shutter speed on a camera. If the motion of the eye or the scene is slow then each photoreceptor output provides an accurate estimate of the amount of light in one small scene patch, but if the motion is fast then each photoreceptor output represents a mixture of light intensities associated with the scene points that just whizzed across the photoreceptor. The result is that each image point effectively gets smeared out across many photoreceptors, giving rise to the blur apparent in many photographs.

Shape from Motion
Just as motion parallax can tell us the distances to points in a scene if we are moving, so it can also tell us the distances to points on an object if the object is moving. In the case of an object, knowing these distances effectively specifies the object's three-dimensional shape. In particular, if an object is rotating, even by a small amount, then the relative speeds *in the retinal image* of nearby features *on the object* are determined by their relative distances, and therefore give some idea of the 3-D shape of the object.

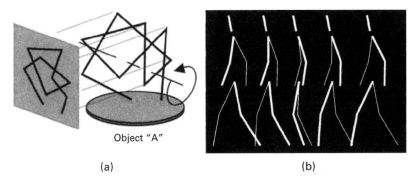

Object "A"

(a)   (b)

Figure 5.15
Kinetic depth effect. (a) Three-dimensional rigid wire-frame object is rocked back and forth around a vertical axis between ±20 degrees, and its image is projected onto a screen. Observing the sequence of two-dimensional images on the screen gives a compelling impression of a three-dimensional object. (b) Consecutive frames from a screen sequence obtained by rotating a rigid wire-frame matchstick figure back and forth around its vertical axis gives the impression of a person walking. Reproduced from Sinha and Poggio 1996.

An elegant demonstration of the power of motion to specify three-dimensional shape is given by the *kinetic depth effect*, shown in figure 5.15a. A rigid wire is first bent into a complex 3-D shape, and a light is used to project an image of the wire on to a screen. If the wire is static then it's very difficult to make out any particular three-dimensional shape by looking at the screen, but as soon as the wire begins to rotate, the resultant sequence of two-dimensional shapes on the screen immediately gives the impression of the correct 3-D shape. This is a prime example of how the visual system extracts *structure from motion* (also called *shape from motion*). However, if the wire-frame object doesn't contain any sharp turns but curves smoothly then the screen sequence can easily be misinterpreted as an object that deforms over time.

A key assumption required to estimate the three-dimensional structure of an object from its motion is that the object is rigid, that it doesn't change its 3-D shape during motion. For many years, it was thought that the human visual system makes this *rigidity assumption*, except in the case of the "curved-wire" objects described in the last paragraph.

Then, in 1996, Pawan Sinha and Tomaso Poggio provided a perfect counter-example. They rotated a wire-frame object through ±20 degrees around a vertical axis to give the impression of a three-dimensional shape when projected onto a screen, as shown in figure 5.15. Let's call this "object

X." After experimental observers viewed screen sequences from object X for some time, it was replaced with 3-D object Y, specifically designed to be similar to object X, so that both X and Y gave the same two-dimensional screen shape when they were at the midpoint of their rotating motion. However, because the 3-D shape of Y was similar, but not identical, to the object X, it gave rise to a different sequence of 2-D shapes on the screen when it was rotated.

Sinha and Poggio reasoned that observers not previously exposed to object X would perceive object Y correctly, as a *rigid* 3-D wire-frame object, whereas those previously exposed would misperceive object Y as object X. And this proved to be the case. That is, when observers previously exposed to object X saw the 2-D screen sequence generated by a different object (Y), they misidentified it as a "bendy" version of object X.

The study dealt a coup de grâce to the rigidity assumption when Sinha and Poggio rotated rigid wire-frame matchstick figures (figure 5.15b) around a vertical axis. Their observers perceived the two-dimensional screen projections of these matchstick figures not as *rigid* three-dimensional shapes but as flexible ones of people walking. In other words, after many years of seeing people walk, the brain interprets the sequence of two-dimensional human shapes projected from rigid three-dimensional ones as doing what human figures normally do: walking.

Researchers had known since the early 1970s that we tend to perceive anything that could possibly be a person walking as if it were, in fact, a person walking. Gunnar Johansson (1973) took movies of humans walking, and then stripped out everything except for eleven dots, with each dot attached to a major joint, such as an elbow. Seen in isolation, a single frame from a Johansson movie looks like eleven dots, which, depending on the frame, could conceivably be a person, as shown in figure 5.16. But when the frames are seen as a sequence then it is almost impossible not to immediately see a human walking. Indeed, these minimal stimuli can be used to portray the most complex human actions, and they can also portray animals, which are identified with surprising accuracy.

Centuries before Johansson published these results in 1973, William Shakespeare had noted through his character Cassius how the identity of an individual can be gleaned from the way he walks: "'Tis Cinna, I do know him by his gait" (*Julius Caesar*, 1.3.2). Although researchers haven't tested this insight in the laboratory, George Mather and Linda Murdoch (1994) have established that the gender of figures in Johansson movies can be identified from their characteristic movements. Thus motion tells us not only about the structure of entire scenes, but also about objects in

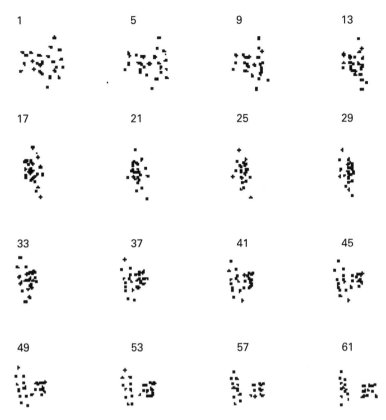

Figure 5.16
Walking the dog. Numbered frames from a Johansson movie of a man walking his dog.

motion; indeed, people in motion betray not only their gender, but perhaps even their identity.

How Much Structure from How Much Motion?

Before leaving the topic of structure from motion, we should establish precisely what information motion conveys, at least in principle, about the structure of an object (figure 5.17). We can reduce the general problem for a brain or a machine of obtaining three-dimensional structure from a sequence of views to the following bare essentials. If an object is rotated a little so that most of the points on its surface remain in view, then three views are sufficient for observers to estimate the three-dimensional structure of that surface, provided observers can match up at least four different

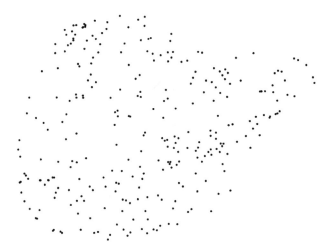

Figure 5.17
Three-dimensional structure of the surface on this object can be obtained from the frames of a motion sequence.

points between the three views. Shimon Ullman (1979) obtained a related result based on four points from three views. His finding follows in a mathematical tradition that can be traced back to a breakthrough requiring five matched points in two views by Erwin Kruppa (1913).

The condition that observers need to "match up" corresponding points in different views equates to knowing which point has moved to where between views, and is known as the "correspondence problem." In essence, if you know how far each of at least four points has moved across your retina between three views of a rotating object then you can estimate the three-dimensional structure of its surface.

Of course, when you see an object, you usually have access to many more than three views (e.g., if you walk past it or rotate it manually), and you can presumably identify many more than four corresponding points between views. However, experimental results reviewed by James T. Todd (1995) indicate that having access to more than two views does not improve the accuracy with which observers perceive three-dimensional shape. Even so, it's interesting to note that a computational analysis of the problem of structure from motion tells us that exactly three views *ought* to be sufficient.

Stereo Vision

In the country of the blind, the one-eyed man is king.

—Desiderius Erasmus, *Adagia*

For those of us with stereo vision, seeing depth seems unremarkable. But if you've spent most of your life without stereo vision then you can fully appreciate the impact of acquiring it. This is what happened to Dr. Susan Barry, who was stereoblind from infancy, due to a squint. In adulthood, she was able to learn to acquire stereo vision, and her reaction tells of the profound difference it made to her how she saw the world:

> I got the powerful sense of being immersed in a three-dimensional world that I never experienced before. . . . Before, if I looked at a snowfall, the snowflakes appeared a little distance away from me in one flat plane. When I gained stereo vision, I felt myself within the snowfall: the snow was falling all around me in many levels of depth. (Barry 2009).

It seems self-evident that having two eyes is better than having one. If this really were the case then, surely, having three eyes would be better than having two? Indeed, there are creatures with more, and fewer, than two eyes. Many crustaceans have only one eye, jumping spiders have eight, and the humble scallop has hundreds. But, as always, there are both costs and benefits to having more than one eye. Each extra eye has to be grown during development, fed with nutrients, and maintained throughout life. In other words, the Darwinian fitness benefits must outweigh the various costs that each extra eye demands.

Having two eyes enables prey animals like rabbits to see almost all around them: each eye has a large field of view, and there is almost no overlap between the views of their two eyes. Having two eyes with overlapping views allows predators, such as an eagle (figure 5.18) or an owl

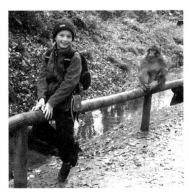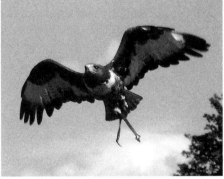

Figure 5.18
Forward-facing eyes of humans, monkeys, and eagles ensure they have good stereo vision.

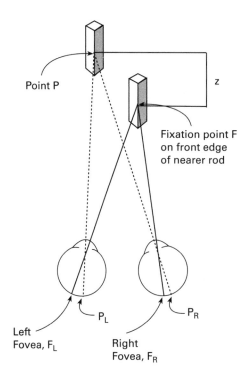

Point P

z

Fixation point F
on front edge
of nearer rod

P_L

P_R

Left
Fovea, F_L

Right
Fovea, F_R

Figure 5.19
Geometric origin of stereo disparity. If the eyes fixate on a three-dimensional point
F in the world then the image of this point falls on the left fovea F_L, and also on
the right fovea F_R. A different three-dimensional point, P, falls on a point P_L in the
left eye, a distance of v_L millimeters away from the left fovea F_L, and it falls on a
point P_R in the right eye, v_R millimeters from the right fovea F_R. The difference
between the distances v_L and v_R is the stereo disparity of the 3-D point P, and can
be used to find the depth interval z. From Frisby & Stone 2010.

(van der Willigen 2011), to estimate depth with great accuracy using stereo
vision, or *stereopsis* as it's known (figure 5.19).

One way to think about stereopsis is as a form of "simultaneous" motion
parallax (figure 5.20). You can consider the two different views obtained
by your left and right eyes as the first and final frames of a sequence during
which your left eye moves to where your right eye is, and generates an
optic flow field in the process. The structure of this vector field is identical
whether based on two images from a single eye at two points in space and
time (i.e., through motion) or on two images from two eyes at different
positions but at the same time (i.e., through stereopsis).

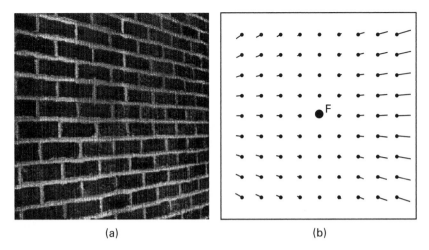

(a)   (b)

Figure 5.20
Stereo disparities. (a) Plane receding in depth. (b) Stereo disparities in the cyclopean image associated with different points on the slanted plane in (a) and generated by looking at the center of the plane. The fixation point F corresponds to the three-dimensional point on the plane that both eyes are looking at. Each dot represents the position of a 3-D point in the left eye's view, and the end of each dot's line represents the position of the same 3-D point in the right eye's view. The result is an optic flow field that would be obtained if the left eye moved to where the right eye is. Note that the "arrows" point in opposite directions on the left and right side of the cyclopean image, implying a change in the direction of travel for near and far points. From Frisby & Stone 2010.

A more mathematical way of exploring stereopsis goes like this. Because your eyes are separated by a few centimeters, each eye has a different view of the world, so that your two retinal images are slightly different. The point in a scene that your eyes are looking at, the *fixation point F*, projects to the center of the fovea F_L in your left eye, and the center of the fovea F_R in your right eye. As shown in figure 5.19, another three-dimensional point P projects to a point P_L in your left eye, and to a point P_R in your right eye. Crucially, the distance between F_L and P_L in your left eye is different from the distance between F_R and P_R in your right. For example, this distance might be $v_L = 0.1$ mm in your left eye, but $v_R = 0.3$ mm in your right. The difference between these distances depends on the depth of the three-dimensional point P, and defines the *retinal disparity* between the image points P_L and P_R, which in this case is $v_L - v_R = 0.1$ mm $- 0.3$ mm $= -0.2$ mm. In practice, each of these quantities is expressed, not as a distance across the retina, but in terms of an equivalent optic angle (see p. 57).

Note that every point in a three-dimensional scene projects to a single point in each of your retinal images. If these two images are overlaid then we obtain a *cyclopean image* ("cyclopean" after the one-eyed giant of Homer's *Odyssey*), as shown in figure 5.20b. The image is assumed to be centered on a point mid-way between your eyes—the cyclopean center. Within this image, the difference between each pair of corresponding retinal points defines a small directed line that connects them. Thus each line is actually an arrow or *vector* that specifies how a single point in the left image moves to a corresponding point in the right image. These lines collectively define a *vector field*, which is similar to the flow field obtained when considering structure from motion or motion parallax.

As we shall see shortly, stereo disparity provides us not with *absolute* depth, but with the depth of points *relative* to the fixation point. This makes sense because the disparity of the fixation point is, by definition, zero. The retinal disparity of another three-dimensional point P increases as it moves away from the fixation point. The difference between the depth of the fixation point and the depth of the point P is called the "depth interval" of P, and is denoted by the letter z.

Consider a pair of eyes separated by a typical distance of $I = 6$ cm that are looking at the fixation point F, which has a depth d, and another point P with a depth interval z. The disparity H of P is the distance between the projections of P into the left and right eyes' images (see figure 5.19). The disparity, measured in degrees, is given by the *disparity equation*:

$H = cIz/d^2$ degrees,

where the constant $c = 57.3$ degrees/radian (and ensures that H is expressed in degrees rather than in radians.) However, because the visual system is very sensitive to disparity, H is often expressed in terms of minutes (60 minutes in one degree) or seconds (60 seconds in one minute). This equation is included here for two reasons.

First, using stereopsis, retinal disparity tells the brain the absolute depth of points only if it knows is the distance d to the fixation point. Without this information, the brain only knows which points are nearer or farther than the fixation point, but not how much nearer or farther. This means that stereopsis may only give a rough idea of three-dimensional shape, one that simply ranks the relative depth of points. This, in turn, suggests that a world stretched along your line of sight (i.e., along the z-axis) would look pretty much the same to you as one compressed along your line of sight. Indeed, this prediction was found to be accurate when Andrew Glennerster and colleagues (2006) tested it experimentally using a virtual reality device.

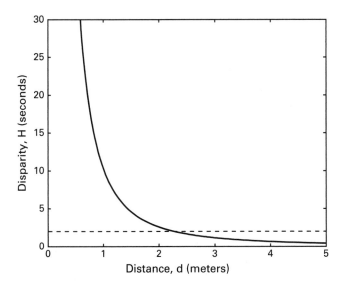

Figure 5.21
Graph showing how retinal disparity H decreases with distance for a fixed depth
interval of $z = 1$ centimeter. The dashed line indicates the threshold of human stereo
perception (2 arc seconds). This implies that a 1-centimeter cube provides no detectable stereo disparity beyond a distance of about 2.5 meters.

The second reason for presenting the disparity equation above is to
show how mathematics enables us to work out what can be achieved by
the brain in a principled manner. It's often claimed that stereopsis ceases
to be of any use beyond a few meters. This claim appears to be supported
by the graph in figure 5.21, which shows how the stereo disparity of a
1-centimeter die decreases as its distance from the eyes increases. Given
that the threshold for human stereopsis is about 2 arc seconds (Coutant
& Westheimer 1993), this implies that stereopsis can't provide information about shape (i.e., depth interval) once the die is farther than about
2.5 meters away. However, a bigger object at any given distance provides
larger stereo disparities, and the disparity equation can be used to find
out exactly how big these disparities are for a given object size. For
example, one side of New York's Chrysler Building is about $z = 300$ meters
wide, and when it is viewed edge-on from a distance of 450 meters (about
a quarter mile), the depth interval z gives rise to a just-detectable disparity
of 2 arc seconds. Obviously, distances less than 450 meters yield disparities
increasingly easy to detect, which therefore give an increasingly strong
impression of the three-dimensional structure of the building. The point

is that, once the disparity equation is understood, we are not mystified when we find experimentally that stereopsis provides almost no information about the three-dimensional structure of a 1-centimeter cube at a distance greater than 2.5 meters. The math tells us that such a situation yields almost no stereo disparity, and so no vision system (biological or otherwise) could possibly perceive the cube's 3-D structure using stereopsis under these circumstances. Similarly, the math tells us that widely spaced eyes should yield more disparity, and therefore more depth information, than eyes that are close together. More importantly, the math tells us precisely *how much* depth perception should improve for every extra millimeter added to the distance between the eyes. Indeed, preliminary results by my colleague John Frisby and others suggest that top sports performers tend to have widely spaced eyes. In the animal kingdom, the hammerhead shark, shown in figure 5.22b has a hammer for a head which ensures that both eyes' views overlap by 48 degrees (compared to 120 degrees for humans). Even though direct evidence for stereopsis in sharks is lacking, there seems little point in having two views of the same object (e.g., prey) unless these views are combined to obtain 3-D information (McComb et al. 2009). Similarly, the stalk-eyed fly shown in figure 5.22a may have such astonishingly long eye-stalks to ensure accurate depth perception.

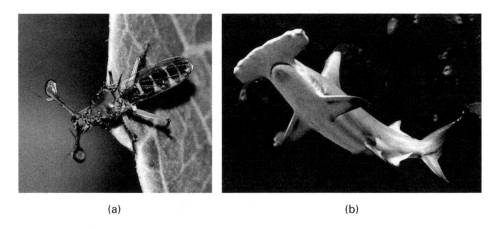

(a)   (b)

Figure 5.22
(a) Male stalk-eyed flies (Diopsidae) have eyes up to 5.5 cm apart with overlapping fields of view, which could mean they have stereoscopic vision. Photograph by Hauke Koch from *Wikipedia*. (b) Hammerhead shark has superb depth perception because its eyes are far apart.

Stereograms

If you placed a camera in front of each of your eyes then the resultant pair of pictures would be a *stereogram*. In other words, a stereogram is a pair of pictures, each of which shows the image from one eye's viewpoint, as in figure 5.23. To see the depth in a stereogram, it is necessary to get one image into the left eye and the other into the right eye. This can be achieved using a stereogram viewer invented by Charles Wheatstone in 1838, colored glasses, or (more recently) polarized light. However, a cheaper method called "free fusion" requires only a pencil or a matchstick and a little patience ("fusion" refers to the fact that two images are fused into a single three-dimensional percept), as shown in figure 5.24. Here is how to do it.

Begin by looking at a point midway between the two stereogram images in figure 5.25, and then place a matchstick about halfway between your eyes and the page. Because you're looking at the page and not the matchstick, you'll see two images of the matchstick, one superimposed over the left image, and the other superimposed over the right image in figure 5.25. Adjust the depth of the matchstick so that each matchstick image appears over the middle of one of the stereogram images. Now—and this is the crucial part—look at the matchstick. When you do this, the center of the left stereogram image ends up in the fovea of your right eye, and the center of the right stereogram image ends up in the fovea of your left eye. Move the matchstick back and forth a little, and then wait. Your visual

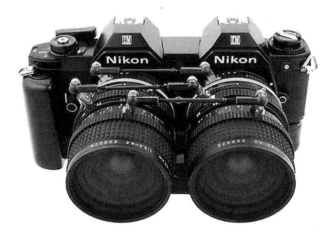

Figure 5.23
Stereo camera made by Max Pow. Reproduced with permission.

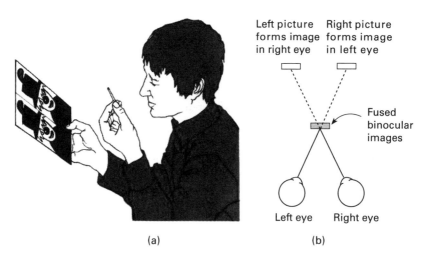

(a)   (b)

Figure 5.24
Free fusion, so called because the images in the two eyes can be fused without any apparatus. (a) How to free-fuse a stereogram. (b) Optics of free fusion. From Frisby & Stone 2010.

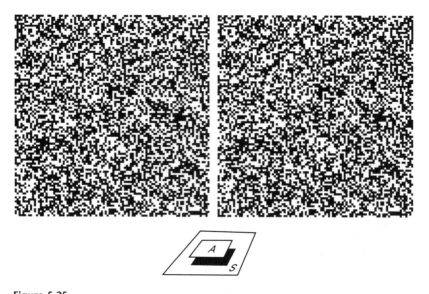

Figure 5.25
Random-dot stereogram. When viewed using free fusion (see figure 5.24), a small square patch (A) appears to float above the surround (S), as depicted in the bottom figure. From Frisby & Stone 2010.

system needs time to lock onto the correct correspondence between points in your left and right eyes' images. You may see a series of diagonal lines forming as your visual system searches out the correct matches. Be patient. Within a minute or so, a sharply defined square hovering above a background should appear. When this happens, slowly move the matchstick down and out of view, while looking at the stereograms. You should now be able to move your eyes about to explore the square floating in space. This method does require some perseverance and concentration, but the results are quite stunning. Next try the free-fusion technique on figure 5.26 or skip ahead to 5.28. Once you've mastered it, you'll be able to view 3-D scenes in the many stereograms available online (especially on websites like flickr.com).

The use of stereograms played a vital role in aerial reconnaissance in the First and Second World Wars. Unlike normal photographs, stereo pairs of photographs made taller structures stand out, so artillery emplacements, munitions factories, and anti-aircraft batteries became relatively easy to detect. This is the feature that allows stereograms to break the camouflage of objects that would otherwise be almost undetectable, as in figure 5.26.

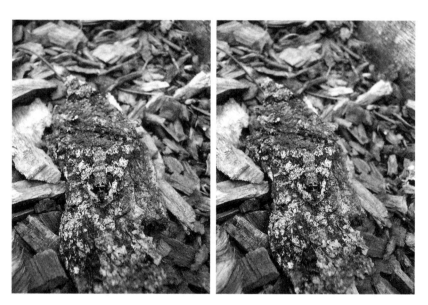

Figure 5.26
Breaking camouflage. This feathered ranunculus moth (*Polymixis lichenea*) is almost invisible in each image, but stands out in depth when viewed stereoscopically.

The Correspondence Problem

All of the above depends on one key assumption: that the brain knows how to match up corresponding points in the left and right images, as shown in figure 5.27. This is a hard problem because the total number of possible *pairwise* matches is $4 \times 4 = 16$, as shown in figure 5.27b. However, the total number of all possible ways to match up all four points in one image with all four points in the other is much larger than sixteen. For example, one *set* of possible four pairwise matches is shown by the four dark disks in figure 5.27b (which happens to represent the correct set of matches). However, any other set of four disks in figure 5.27b also represents a legitimate set of four pairwise matches. Therefore, the number of possible sets of matches is the same as the number of ways that four out of sixteen disks in figure 5.27b can be chosen. Incidentally, choosing four pairwise matches in this way ensures that each point in the left image is paired with exactly one point in the right image, and vice versa. It turns out that there are a total of $4 \times 3 \times 2 \times 1$ or 4! (four *factorial*) = 24 ways to choose four out of the sixteen disks in figure 5.27b. And of those twenty-

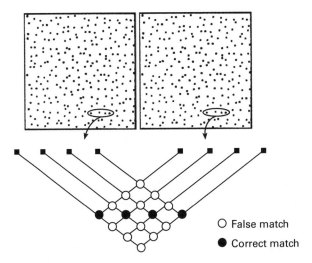

Figure 5.27
Stereo correspondence problem. (a) Each point in the left image must be matched with its corresponding point in the right image. Here points are made explicit as dots, and four dots are encircled to exemplify how many ways they can be (mis-) matched across the two images. (b) Expanded view shows that each dot in the left image can be matched with four dots in the right image (and vice versa), but only one of these matches is correct (black disks), the rest are mismatches (white disks). From Frisby & Stone 2010.

four ways to match up four pairs of points between the left and right images, twenty-three are wrong (Mallot, 2000, p. 133).

More generally, if we consider N image points in the left image, and N in the right image then there are $N!$ possible sets of N pairwise matches, of which $N! - 1$ are wrong. Of course, the number of points in each image can be extremely large. But even if it's as small as 100 then the number of possible matches is 10^{158} (1 followed by 158 zeros). For comparison, there are 10^{80} fundamental particles in the universe. If each point is the output of a photoreceptor, of which there are 126 million in each retinal image then the number of all possible matches is so large it can't be calculated on a modern computer using standard numerical software.

What if the brain first analyses each image for a few salient features (like a stick in figure 5.26) and then tries to match these across the two images? Surely, that would reduce the number of possible matches enormously. Indeed, it used to be thought that this was how the brain solved the correspondence problem. After all, it seems ridiculous to expect the brain to try to match up every visual detail in a typical pair of retinal images, especially because more details imply many more possible matches.

Then, in the late 1950s, Bela Julesz invented the *random-dot stereogram*, an example of which is shown in figure 5.25. This seemed to provide a stark and compelling disproof of the hypothesis that the brain does stereopsis by first finding salient features, which it then uses as a basis for matching.

The essential property of a random-dot stereogram is that the left and right images, when viewed in isolation, look like pure chaos. And each image is indeed constructed by coloring each small square (dot) either black or white at random, so each image really is chaotic. For the example shown in figure 5.25, both left and right images are the same chaos, with one small difference between them. The square patch you see in 3-D corresponds to a square patch of the left image that has been moved a few pixels to the right, so this square patch ends up in a different place in your left and right retinal images. When you look at the images using free fusion, the difference in the positions of this square patch in the left and right images produces a retinal disparity that fools your brain into signaling the presence of a square patch that has a different *depth* from its background. Thus the fact that you can see depth in random-dot stereograms seems to prove that your brain can find the correct set of matches, even when there are no salient features apparent in each image when viewed in isolation. This is like finding a needle in a haystack of $N!$ possible sets of matches.

However, even though the brain doesn't seem to perform stereopsis on the basis of perceptually salient features (like chairs or faces), recent evidence suggests that it matches coarse elements before fine details (Neri 2011). If the matches between coarse elements are used to guide the matches between fine details, then this reduces the magnitude of the correspondence problem enormously. Note that these coarse elements correspond to low spatial frequencies, whereas fine details correspond to high spatial frequencies. In principle, this coarse-to-fine strategy could work even for random-dot stereograms because simple cells with large receptive fields effectively ignore the fine spatial structure of images (as in figure 5.25), and their outputs could be used as a basis for stereo matches at a coarse spatial scale. These matches could then be used to guide the matching of finer spatial scales using the outputs of cells having smaller receptive fields. For example, the random-dot stereogram shown in figure 5.25 is represented in figure 5.28 as the outputs of cells with large receptive fields, which effectively remove all fine details. Despite this, both stereograms convey the same three-dimensional depth information, and both depict a well-defined square shape when viewed with free fusion (see figure 5.24). Indeed, the images in figure 5.28 seem to be easier to fuse, probably because, having fewer image features (i.e., blurred dots) than figure 5.25, they necessarily contain many fewer false matches.

In summary, we seem to have almost come full circle on the correspondence problem. Although the early hypothesis that stereopsis used perceptually salient features to guide the matching of fine details was clearly

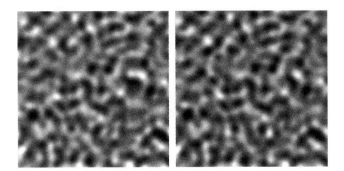

Figure 5.28
Random-dot stereogram shown in figure 5.25, as represented by the outputs of model ganglion cells. Even though most of the fine details (high spatial frequencies) have been removed, the two images can still be fused to reveal the same depth information as in figure 5.25.

disproved by Julesz's random-dot stereograms, it seems that matching large features (whether or not they are perceptually salient) between left and right images might be used as a guide for matching fine features, where the large features would correspond to low spatial frequencies, and fine features to high spatial frequencies.

3-D Glasses

Cinematic 3-D films require the use of two movie cameras: a left camera to take the images from the left eye's point of view and a right camera to take the images from the right eye's point of view. The only remaining problem is how to ensure that, when the film is shown in the movie theater, the left eye sees only images taken by the left camera, and the right eye sees only images taken by the right camera. This is the central conundrum that has faced 3-D cinematography since the first stereo movie cameras were invented.

The earliest attempt at solving this conundrum involved re-coloring the left camera's movie in shades of green, and the right camera's movie in shades of red. The two movies were then shown together, which looked like a visual mess when viewed normally. However, if a green filter is placed over the left eye then the red movie (from the right camera) is almost invisible to the left eye, so only the movie from the left camera can be seen by the left eye. Similarly, a red filter placed over the right eye ensures that only the movie from the right camera can be seen by the right eye. Each movie is thus seen by the correct eye, the brain fuses the images from both movies, and 3-D cinematography was born. But it had a short life, mainly because re-coloring movies in red and green drastically reduces any color information in the original movie.

More recently, 3-D cinematography has been reborn in full color. Its latest incarnation ensures that the light associated with the two images is polarized along two perpendicular directions. When wearing polarizing glasses, each lens accepts light polarized in one orientation only, so that each eye sees the image from one of the stereo cameras only. This method is quite ingenious and has an exact physical analogy to the way that two stereo sound channels were encoded in a single groove in a phonograph record.

Shape from Texture and Shading

The shape of a three-dimensional object can be inferred from its texture or from its shading. The methods that can be used to perform these

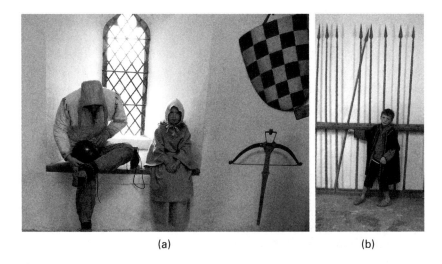

(a)   (b)

Figure 5.29
How easily we are fooled. (a) The girl and the window are real; the man is a dummy; the crossbow and the shield have been painted onto the wall with cleverly placed shadows. The changing shapes of the "square" texture elements in the image of the shield indicate its curvature. (b) Photograph of a wall with spears painted on it; painted shadows give a realistic impression of depth (the boy is real).

inferences, either by the brain or on a computer are called "shape from texture" and "shape from shading." Of course, once the brain accepts that texture and shading are associated with particular changes in an image then it is bound to be fooled from time to time, as in figure 5.29.

Texture and shading represent complementary visual cues; they each act as a powerful cue to the three-dimensional shape of individual objects. For example, the hat shown in figure 5.30 is clearly more shaded on its left-hand side, and the small bumps and dips in the material are demarcated by local changes in shading. Similarly, the changes in texture in the image indicate how the surface orientation changes across the object.

Shape from Texture
The circular disks that pepper the material in figure 5.30 indicate three-dimensional shape in two ways. First, their shapes in the image change as the slant of the material changes. Specifically, the disks appear as circular only for parts of the hat facing the camera, but as the material slants away, so the *circular* disks on the *hat* yield increasingly *elliptical* texture elements in the *image*. Thus, provided the texture elements have a roughly circular

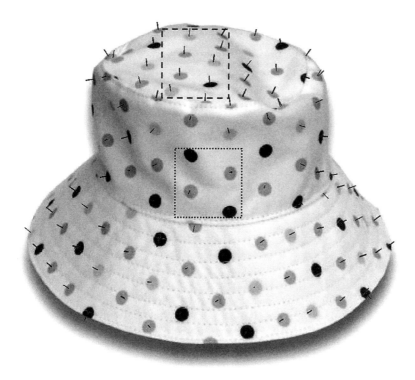

Figure 5.30
Shape from texture and shading. The two squares have identical areas on the page, and show how the number of disks per square centimeter of image area increases with surface slant. Courtesy Angeline Loh (2006).

shape on the surface, the brain or a computer can use their shape in the image to estimate 3-D shape. Textures that have circular texture elements are said to be "isotropic," and one of the first successful shape-from-texture computer programs made use of a general form of the isotropic assumption to find shape from texture.

Second, the number of disks in each small image region varies across the image. The two square outlines in figure 5.30 have the same area on the page, but there are nine disks in the upper dashed square, whereas there are only four in the lower dotted square. Notice that the number of disks in each square centimeter of the material on the hat is constant (i.e., *homogenous*). Therefore, the change in the density of disks in the image is due to the increased slant of the material in different parts of the hat. Thus, provided the texture density is the same everywhere, or *homogeneous*, on the surface, the brain or a computer can use changes in image texture density to estimate three-dimensional shape, just as they can use density to estimate the orientation of the planar surface in figure 5.4.

Crucially, both shape and density change systematically with surface orientation, and the brain or a computer can therefore use them to estimate the local surface orientation of every patch within an image (although they can't use texture to estimate distance because each texture element could be small and near on a small hat, or big and far on a giant hat). If we know the orientation of every patch on an object, by definition, then we also know its overall shape. These cues therefore provide a principle for estimating shape from texture. Indeed, the "needles" sticking out of the hat in figure 5.30 were placed in the image by a computer program that used the shape of individual texture elements to estimate the surface orientation in different regions of the image.

Shape from Shading
Shading clearly gives a strong indication as to the local orientation of a surface, as shown in figure 5.31a. But there is a catch. Any local image darkening could be due to a change in shading (and therefore to a change in surface orientation) or to a change in the proportion of light reflected of the surface (see p. 49).

The perceived *lightness* of a surface is determined by at least three factors. First, the surface is intrinsically light or dark. This is its *albedo*, which is defined as the proportion of light reflected from a surface (see "Luminance"

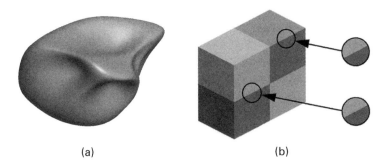

(a)   (b)

Figure 5.31
(a) To obtain shape from shading, you first have to discount the reflectance or albedo of the surface. (b) Lightness illusion. The same change in image luminance (gray level) can be induced either by a change in surface orientation of a surface with constant reflectance (top circle), or by a change in the reflectance of a surface with constant orientation (bottom circle). Courtesy Ted Adelson.

in chapter 3). For example, in figure 5.31b, the surface's albedo, but not its orientation, changes within the lower circle, so the change in luminance (gray level) within the circle is due only to a change in surface albedo. Second, the orientation of a local surface patch with respect to an observer affects the luminance within the corresponding image of that surface patch. In figure 5.31b, the surface's orientation, but not its albedo, changes within the upper circle, so the change in image luminance within the image circle is due only to a change in surface orientation.

Figure 5.31b shows how the same image gray levels can be produced either by a change in albedo with no change in surface orientation (lower circle) or by a change in surface orientation with no change in albedo (upper circle). Even though identical image changes are produced by two different physical scenarios, your visual system isn't fooled into getting the two interpretations of these image patches mixed up. Of course, if you viewed both patches isolated from their image context then there'd be no way to tell them apart because they're identical on the page. Thus the image context somehow allows you to conclude which image changes are due to surface albedo changes and which are due to surface orientation changes. Conversely, you can see the lighter parts of the image in figure 5.31a as reflections of the light source, known as "specularities," rather than as changes in albedo or in surface orientation.

From the above example, it should be apparent that, in order to be able to make use of changes in image gray level to estimate shape, it is necessary to know which gray-level changes are due to changes in surface orientation (i.e., shading), albedo, and specularities. However, because a change in image gray level is usually caused by a combination of all three factors, to estimate shape from shading, the brain needs to separate out or *decompose* the effects of shape, albedo, and specularities on image gray levels, as shown in figures 5.32 and 5.33. As with shape from texture, provided the image gray level changes *systematically* with changes in surface orientation, it is possible to use it to estimate surface orientation or shape from shading, even though the estimated shape is subject to the same type of convexity ambiguity described above for shaded images of faces. Thus, shape from shading provides a rank ordering of points in depth, without specifying the depth of any single point on an object.

Conclusion

Using the visual cues of optic flow, motion parallax, stereopsis, texture, and shading, the brain can recover information that is merely implicit in

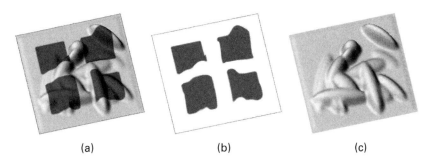

(a)   (b)   (c)

Figure 5.32
Separating the effects of shape and albedo on image gray levels. (a) Bumps are visible mainly because they produce shading differences across the image. However, the image gray level at any one point is determined by a combination of the local surface orientation and by its albedo. To us, it is obvious that there are four square patches with the same dark albedo. (b) With the effects of shape on image gray level removed, the four patches are made explicit. (c) With the effects of albedo on image gray level removed, only the effects of shading remain. Reproduced with permission from Marshall Tappen.

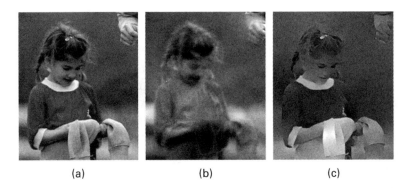

(a)   (b)   (c)

Figure 5.33
Separating out the effects of albedo and shading on image gray levels. Results from a computer program. (a) Original image. (b) Estimated shading information only. (c) Estimated albedo only. Reproduced with permission from Marshall Tappen.

the retinal images. It can use these visual cues to recover different information under different conditions. For example, it can use motion parallax to estimate the three-dimensional structure of an object seen from different views (e.g., resulting from object rotation), and shading information to find the relative depth of different points on the object from a single view.

Additionally, these various cues are more or less reliable depending on the specific conditions. For example, texture cues become increasingly informative as the slant of a surface increases, whereas the information conveyed by stereo disparity is almost immune to slant, but disparity becomes less informative as the distance to a surface increases. To arrive at a reliable conclusion about the shape of a particular object, the brain takes account of the changing reliability of information from different cues (e.g., Knill & Saunders 2003). This is a problem ideally suited to Bayesian inference, a topic we will explore in some detail in the next chapter.

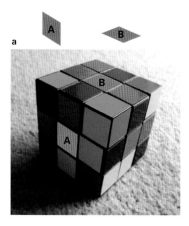

Plate 1 (figure 1.3)
Edited image of a Rubik's cube. The patch labeled A on the side of the cube and the red patch labeled B on the top of the cube share the same color on the printed page, as can be seen when they're shown isolated above the photograph. This illusion was created simply by copying the color of B to A using a graphics application. Based on an illusion by Ted Adelson. From Frisby & Stone 2010.

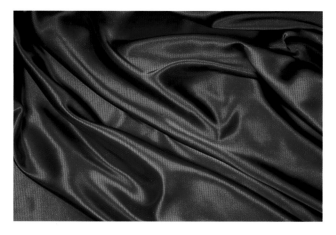

Plate 2 (figure 1.7)
Silk sheet. The three-dimensional shape perceived here is almost entirely due to subtle changes in shading.

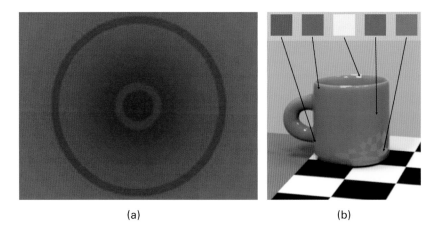

(a)   (b)

Plate 3 (figure 1.11)

Color illusions. A single color at two different locations on the page gives rise to the perception of two different colors in (a), whereas many different colors on the page give rise to the perception of a single color in the world in (b). The square patches at the top of the figure show the colors on the page from the locations indicated by the arrows. Adapted from Xiao & Brainard 2008. Reproduced with permission from MacLeod (2003) and Brainard & Maloney (2011).

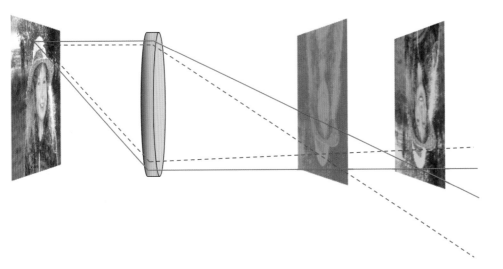

Plate 4 (figure 2.8)

Chromatic aberration. Light reflected from a single point contains a mixture of colors, represented here simply as yellow and blue. Light of different colors gets bent to a different extent, with blue being bent more than yellow. Consequently, if the lens focuses yellow from the subject onto the retina then blue light from the subject forms a perfectly focused image 0.5 mm in front of the retina. This blue light therefore forms a fuzzy image by the time it reaches the retina.

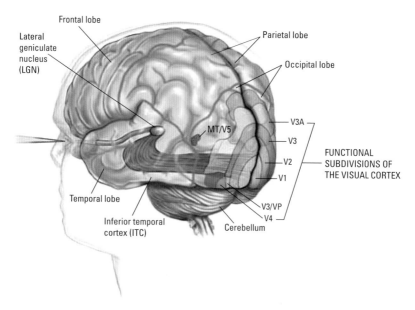

Plate 5 (figure 4.1)

Major divisions of the human brain and visual cortex. Reproduced with permission, copyright © 1999 Terese Winslow.

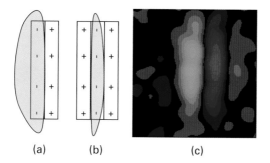

Plate 6 (figure 4.9)

(a, b) Schematic receptive fields of simple cells found in primary visual cortex, with shaded regions showing the approximate pattern of light and dark that yields the maximum response from each cell. The sign (+,–) indicates whether light has an excitatory or inhibitory effect on the simple cell within each region of its receptive field. The two basic types of simple cells are sensitive to (a) luminance edges and (b) lines. Receptive fields with the + and – signs swapped also exist in equal numbers. (c) Color-coded response of a simple cell receptive field, with red showing inhibitory region, and green showing excitatory region. Reproduced with permission.

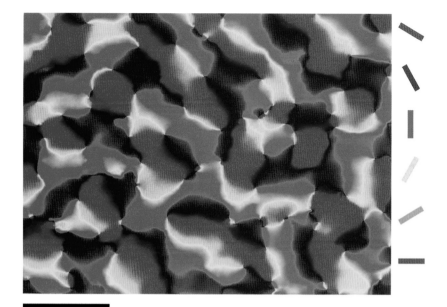

Plate 7 (figure 4.12)
False-color orientation map in primary visual cortex, as viewed from above the cortical surface. The preferred orientation of cells within each cortical area is indicated by color, as shown in the key on the right of the figure. Scale bar: 1 mm. Reproduced with permission from Blasdel 1992.

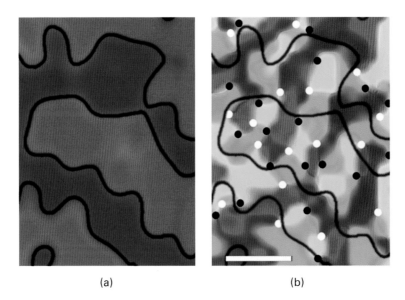

(a)   (b)

Plate 8 (figure 4.16)
Striate cortex as a polymap of different parameters. (a) Human ocularity map. (b) Color-coded orientation map. Both maps cover the same region of human striate cortex, and the black curves in (b) indicate the borders of the ocularity stripes also shown in (a), where dots indicate pinwheels. Obtained using functional magnetic resonance imaging (fMRI). Reproduced with permission from Yacoub, Harel, & Ugurbil 2008, copyright © 2008 National Academy of Sciences, USA.

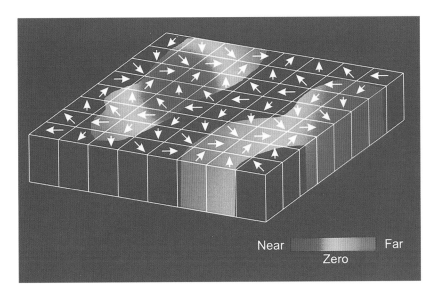

Plate 9 (figure 4.18)
Area MT (V5) codes for motion and stereo disparity. Schematic diagram in which arrows show the preferred direction and color shows the stereo disparity of cells. The terms "near" and "far" refer to the amount of stereo disparity. Reproduced with permission from DeAngelis & Newsome 1999.

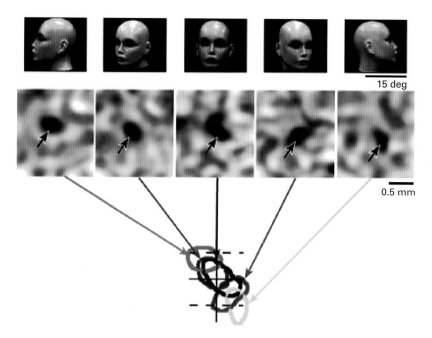

Plate 10 (figure 4.20)

Face-view cells in inferotemporal cortex. The view shown at the top evokes activity in cortex (middle row) at a location shown by the dark spot. The cortical locations of these spots have been overlaid at the bottom to shown how similar views evoke activity in adjacent cortical regions. This suggests that nearby cortical locations represent similar face views. Reproduced with permission from Tanaka 2004; Wang, Tanaka, & Tanifuji 1996.

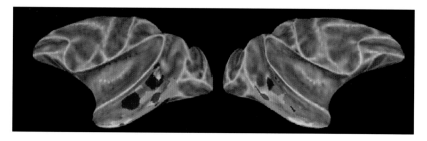

Plate 11 (figure 4.21)

Inflated views of the monkey brain showing regions of inferotemporal cortex selective for faces (red), body parts (yellow), objects (green), and places (blue). Reproduced with permission from Bell et al. 2009.

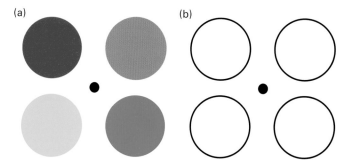

Plate 12 (figure 7.1)
Color aftereffect. (a) Four disks colored red, green, yellow, and blue. (b) Same four disks without color. Fix your gaze on the central black dot in (a) for about 30 seconds, then transfer your gaze to the black dot in (b) and notice the perceived color of the disks. Why does red give a green and blue a yellow aftereffect? From Frisby & Stone 2010.

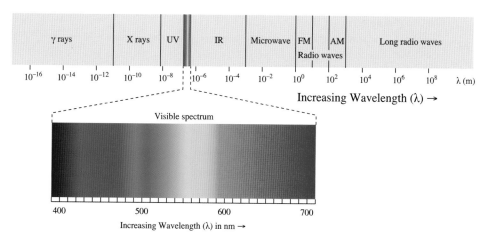

Plate 13 (figure 7.2)
Spectrum of electromagnetic radiation, showing an expanded version of the spectrum's visible part between 400 and 700 nm (where 1,000 nm is a thousandth of a millimeter). Light behaves like a wave, and the distance between consecutive peaks is its wavelength, represented by the Greek letter lambda (λ). Figure by Philip Ronan. Courtesy Creative Commons.

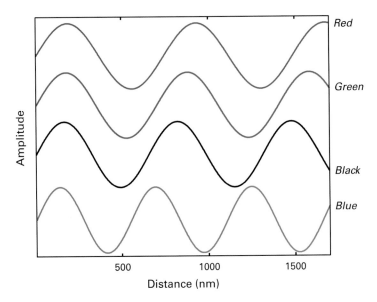

Plate 14 (figure 7.3)
Comparison of wavelengths for retinal photoreceptors. The red curve shows the wavelength (564 nm) of light to which red L-cones are most sensitive, green shows the wavelength (533 nm) to which green M-cones are most sensitive, and blue shows the wavelength (420 nm) to which blue S-cones are most sensitive. The black curve shows the wavelength (498 nm) to which rods are most sensitive.

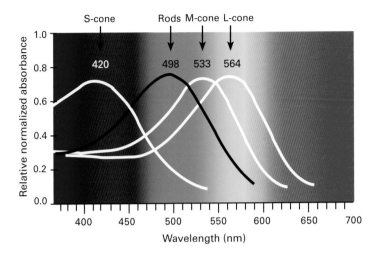

Plate 15 (figure 7.4)
Photoreceptor sensitivity to different wavelengths of light. The sensitivity of each photoreceptor type to different wavelengths of light defines its relative spectral absorbance, or tuning curve. Each curve is the tuning curve of one photoreceptor type. There are three cone types: L (red), M (green) and S (blue). The number above each curve gives the peak sensitivity wavelength in nanometers (nm). Based on data from Bowmaker & Dartnall 1980; reproduced from Frisby & Stone 2010.

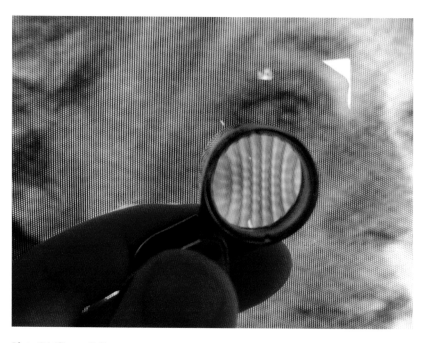

Plate 16 (figure 7.5)
Color television picture consists of a mosaic of triplets of red-, green-, and blue-colored pixels, which can be seen through a magnifying glass. The blue pixels are quite dark here because the underlying picture is of a face, which contains very little blue.

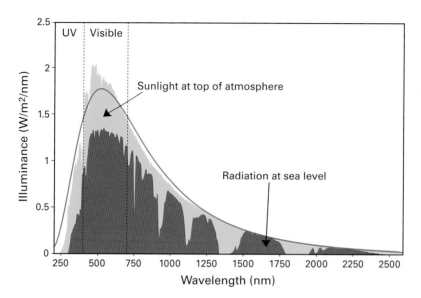

Plate 17 (figure 7.6)

Most terrestrial animals see light with wavelengths between 400 and 700 nm because that's where sunlight's energy peaks. The yellow shading shows which wavelengths dominate at the top of the atmosphere, whereas red shows how much light energy at each wavelength survives sea level. The vertical axis indicates watts (energy per second) per square meter at each wavelength. By RA Rohde, Global Warming Art project, Creative Commons.

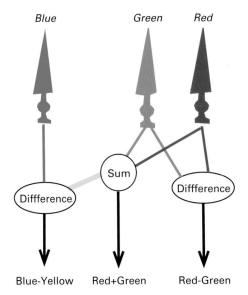

Blue   Green   Red

Sum

Diffference   Diffference

Blue-Yellow   Red+Green   Red-Green

Plate 18 (figure 7.9)
Combining cone outputs to produce three color information channels. The red + green channel is known as the "luminance channel." From Frisby & Stone 2010.

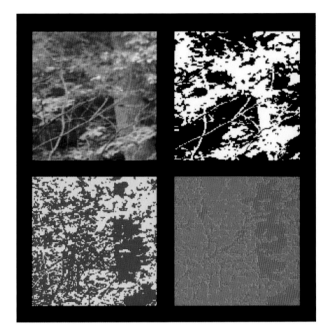

Plate 19 (figure 7.11)
Idealized version of the output of three color channels defined in figure 7.9 (plate 18), based on an original image (top left). The output of the red + green or luminance (upper right), blue – yellow (lower left), and red – green (lower right) channels. Reproduced with permission from Cronin, Ruderman, & Chiao 1998.

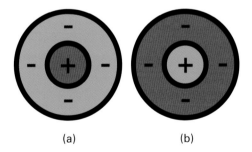

(a) (b)

Plate 20 (figure 7.12)
Schematic diagram of typical receptive fields of red/green center-surround ganglion cells. (a) Red light in the center excites this cell, whereas green in the annulus inhibits it. As the ganglion cell is connected mainly to red-sensitive cones in the center, and mainly to green-sensitive cones in the annulus, this cell shows a spatial red/green opponency, analogous to the luminance opponency shown in figure 3.23. (b) Green light in the center excites this cell, whereas red in the annulus inhibits it.

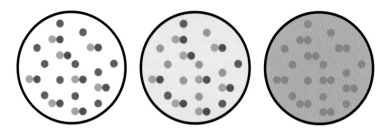

Plate 21 (figure 7.13)

Schematic diagram of typical receptive field of a bistratified retinal ganglion cell, which is excited by blue light and inhibited by yellow light. (Left) Yellow channel is represented by pairs of red and green cones, and the number of blue-sensitive cones is about the same as the combined number of red- and green-sensitive cones in this example. (Middle) Yellow light excites the red/green receptors, which have inhibitory connections to the ganglion cell. (Right) Blue light excites the blue receptors, which have excitatory connections to the ganglion cell.

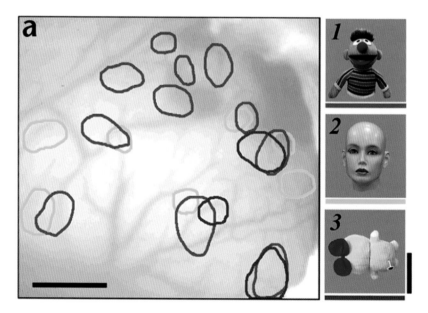

Plate 22 (figure 8.5)

Cells that respond to different objects in area TE, showing spatial distributions of active spots elicited by three different objects. Scale bar in (a): 1 mm.

6 The Perfect Guessing Machine

Seeing is not a direct apprehension of reality, as we often like to pretend. Quite the contrary: *seeing is inference from incomplete information* ...
—E. T. Jaynes, 2003 (p. 133)

Impressions

Your knowledge alters how you see things. The things you see become part of your knowledge. Your knowledge alters how you see things. You can never see the things themselves.

If you were presented with an object that was, in *every* respect, unlike any other object you had ever encountered, what would you see? Nothing? Everything? Or a mixture of every object you have ever seen? But which particular mixture, one based on how prevalent each object was in your past experience?

To take a more realistic example, suppose you were presented with an object, but blurred as if shrouded in thick fog, and then the fog was gradually removed, as in figure 6.1. At first, what you see is dominated by your own personal expectations and beliefs about what the world contains because there is too little information in the retinal image. As the fog becomes thinner, these expectations gradually give way to an increasingly distinct form emerging from the mist. In other words, the influence of your prior expectations on what you perceive diminishes as the fog recedes, and the influence of the image data increases. So, if we are willing to accept that "seeing is believing," then we should also accept that "believing is seeing."

When there is too little information, the brain is forced to replace the missing information with its best guess as to what that information would be. For example, the gradual onset of blindness effectively robs the visual system of information. For a visual system accustomed to receiving

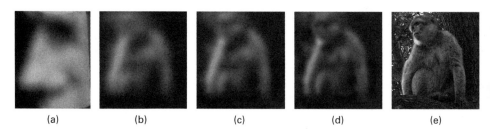

(a)   (b)   (c)   (d)   (e)

Figure 6.1
The influence of our prior expectations on what we perceive becomes more apparent
as image data is degraded. For example, it's easy to interpret the image in (a) as a
nose, perhaps because, for us, noses are a common sight, whereas rhesus monkeys
are less common. The image on the right has been progressively blurred to produce
images (b–d), and (a) is just a close-up of a nose. (a) by Giovanni Lucifero.

high-quality data, the missing data gets replaced by the brain's best guess
at what should be in the retinal image. The result is that people who are
going blind can suffer from *Charles Bonnet syndrome*, which includes visual
hallucinations of animals, houses, and faces, as the brain strives to replace
the missing information. This syndrome usually lasts for several months,
which is presumably how long it takes the visual system to adapt to the
lack of reliable information.

So, what you perceive is based partly on the data that is the retinal
images and partly on your expectations about what the retinal image
should contain, which can be summarized as follows:

perceived image = image data + prior expectations.

This is an informal version of what is probably the single most important equation in probability theory—*Bayes' rule* or *Bayes' theorem*—which
we'll consider in its full form later in this chapter.

Of course, it has long been acknowledged that we rely both on image
data and on our prior expectations to make sense of our retinal images. As
Leonardo da Vinci (1492, in Baltrusatis 1989, p. 61) noted: "If you look at
walls that are stained or made of different kinds of stones . . . you can
think you see in them certain picturesque views of mountains, rivers, rocks,
trees, plains, broad valleys, and hills of different shapes . . . battles and
rapidly moving figures, strange faces and costumes, as well as an infinite
number of things. . . ." Hermann von Helmholtz (1867) often referred to
perception as a process of "unconscious inference," and William James
(1890) once observed: "Whilst part of what we see comes through our
senses from the object before us, another part (and it may be the larger

part) always comes out of our head." More recently, this idea has been eloquently championed by the late Richard Gregory (1997a, 1997b).

However, even though we know that the brain must rely on previous experience, Bayes' rule can inform the brain precisely *how much* it should rely on image data relative to previous experience. The result of combining information from current data (e.g., an image) with information based on experience using Bayes' rule is called "Bayesian inference."

Bayes' rule applies not only to high-level constructs like whole objects, but to any situation in which information is missing. The ubiquitous presence of noise in measurement devices, such as photoreceptors, retinal ganglion cells, or neurons, implies that information, in effect, is always "missing" because it has been corrupted by noise. This in turn implies that Bayes' rule can be used to make "the best of a bad job" by using prior expectations as a proxy for missing information.

However, it is not only mist or noise that impedes perception. The perfectly clear images in figures 1.8, 1.9, 6.2, and 6.5 are also hard to interpret in the absence of basic prior assumptions about lighting direction, 3-D facial structure, and viewpoint, respectively. Even the classic face-vase illusion in figure 6.2 is essentially noise-free, but it can be perceived either as

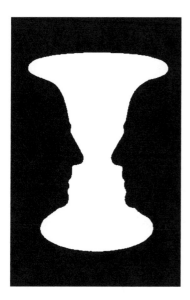

Figure 6.2
Face-vase illusion. Even though this image is free of visual noise, it is still ambiguous and can be perceived either as a pair of faces or as a vase. Reproduced with permission from John Smithson *Wikipedia*.

a pair of faces or as a vase. So Bayes' rule is useful at different levels in the hierarchy of perceptual processing. At the level of individual photoreceptors or neurons, Bayes' rule can be used to find the best estimate of what the underlying noise-free outputs are. When it comes to interpreting images that would be ambiguous even if there were no noise, the use of additional information, for example, in the form of a light-from-above assumption disambiguates the perceived image (e.g., figure 1.8). Thus, even for essentially noise-free data, Bayes' rule allows us to combine data with experience to arrive at a sensible conclusion. For example, a doctor presented with a patient having spots knows that this symptom is equally consistent with two diseases, smallpox and chicken pox. So the probability of the data (spots) given each of the possible diseases is the same (i.e., about 0.99). However, if the doctor brings extra information to bear, in the form of prior experience then he knows that chicken pox is common, and he should know that smallpox was the first human disease to be eradicated in 1979. This prior knowledge allows the doctor to correctly infer that the patient's disease is almost certainly chicken pox. Although this may appear to be plain common sense, it is also an example of Bayesian inference. Additionally, it serves to demonstrate that there is no conflict between common sense reasoning and Bayesian inference.

Perfectly Ambiguous Images

Look at the image in figure 6.3a. Do you see a cube or the inside of a box? Most people first see a cube, but if they keep on looking then the cube suddenly flips and they see it as the inside of a box or a room (which we will call a "box-room" for brevity). The problem that the visual system struggles with here is that the image on the page (and therefore on the retina) does not contain enough information to specify which is the correct three-dimensional interpretation. So the brain keeps changing its mind, first choosing one, then the other interpretation.

From this simple example, and others given in chapter 1, it is apparent that what we see depends on two different sources of information. One of these sources is the retinal image, and the other is the brain's expectations about what dimensional shapes might be in the world. The relative amounts of information from these two sources depend on how reliable the image information is, and on how strong are our expectations about what the retinal image could depict.

In the case of the image in figure 6.3a, the image information is *equally* consistent with a cube and a box-room, so we can define it as being *perfectly*

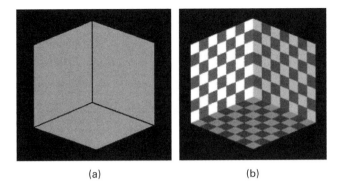

(a)   (b)

Figure 6.3
(a) Perfectly ambiguous image of a 3-D shape can be seen as a convex cube, a concave box-room, or as one of many shallow cube-like structures with different degrees of depth as measured from front to back (which is hard for us to perceive). (b) If the texture on the surface is assumed to consist of squares then there are only two possible 3-D interpretations, a convex cube and a concave box-room.

ambiguous. Images like the one in figure 6.3a make excellent tools for probing how perception works because perfect ambiguity forces the brain to rely on previous experience with similar images in order to guess which three-dimensional interpretation is correct. In contrast, because most natural images are not equally consistent with two 3-D shapes, the brain can use the image information alone to estimate their 3-D shape. However, as we will see, estimates of 3-D shape based both on image data and on previous experience are, on average, more accurate than those based on image data alone.

In order to understand the Bayesian framework, we need to consider the shape of the three-dimensional object in terms of a single quantity or *parameter*. If the object has no surface texture, as in figure 6.3a, then it could be a cube, which is *convex* because it seems to stick out from the page, or a box-room, which is *concave* because it seems to recede into the page. In principle, it could also be seen as perfectly flat, or part-way between flat and convex, or part-way between flat and concave, even though it is difficult for us to see it as these intermediate shapes. Thus the image in figure 6.3a could depict a 3-D shape with any *degree of convexity* between a cube and a box-room. We can define this "degree of convexity" in terms of a single parameter c, where $c = 1$ corresponds to a cube, $c = 0$ corresponds to a flat shape, and $c = -1$ corresponds to a box-room. For example, a value of $c = 0.5$ defines a 3-D shape midway between a flat shape and a cube, that is, a "shallow" cube with only a small amount of depth.

Before continuing, let's review the new terms introduced above. A single *parameter* or *variable c* can adopt any *value*. Note that *convexity c* of any object can be defined as the (signed) difference between the depth of an object at its center and a fixed reference point (e.g., a vertex) on its perimeter. Second, we define two fixed values of the parameter c as $c_0 = +1$ to correspond to a convex shape and $c_1 = -1$ to correspond to a concave one. Finally, for the 3-D shape under consideration, we define c_0 to be the *true value* of the parameter c (i.e., the 3-D shape really is a cube).

How Probable Is That Image?

The image in figure 6.3a could have been generated by a three-dimensional shape with any degree of convexity, from a cube to a box-room to any other 3-D shape with any other value of c. Each of these shapes corresponds to a unique value of the convexity parameter c. So now we can ask the question, which three-dimensional shape and, equivalently, which parameter value c is most likely to have yielded the image observed in figure 6.3a?

We could answer this question by varying the degree of convexity between c_1 (concave) and c_0 (convex), and taking a photograph of the 3-D shape associated with each unique value of c, from the same viewpoint as in figure 6.3a. We could then check the match between each photograph and the observed image in figure 6.3a. However, we would find that *all* of those 3-D shapes would yield exactly the same image as in figure 6.3a. Thus every value of the parameter c gives the same image, which is identical to the observed image (figure 6.3a). In other words, the image data alone is insufficient to allow us to come to a decision regarding the 3-D shape of the object because every 3-D shape considered (and therefore every value of c) yields *exactly* the same image.

This can made more formal if we take a short diversion to introduce the idea of a *conditional probability*. We begin by representing the retinal image (which could be figure 6.3a, for example) as the bold letter **x**. If the object that gives rise to the retinal image has some degree of convexity then (except for the example above) the image observed usually depends on the precise value of the convexity parameter c. The probability that the retinal image is **x** given that the value of the convexity parameter is c is written as $p(\mathbf{x}|c)$, where the vertical bar is read, "given that." The fact that we are actually interested in the probability of different values of c, rather than x, means that $p(x|c)$ is known as the "likelihood" of c. In order to emphasize that it is c that is the quantity of interest, the likelihood $p(x|c)$ can also be written as $L(c|x)$.

We have already established above that we would obtain the *same* image for every value c, so the value of the likelihood $p(x|c)$ is the same for all values of the parameter c. Additionally, even though the image *usually* depends on the convexity parameter c, in this particular case, the image is the same for all values of c, and so the probability $p(x|c)$ of this image is the same for all values of c. We do not actually know the *value* of this probability, but that is not our main concern here.

Note that the image is considered to be some *data* measured in the world, whereas the convexity is considered to be a parameter whose value we seek to estimate, so the generic form for a likelihood is

probability(data|parameter value) = $p(x|c)$.

We can make this more realistic if we allow the three-dimensional shape to have a textured surface, as in figure 6.3b. If we assume that the pattern on the surface of the object contains *squares* then this permits exactly two possible 3-D interpretations, a convex cube and a concave box-room. In contrast, the lack of a surface texture in figure 6.3a is consistent with any degree of convexity. So the presence of a square texture excludes all 3-D interpretations involving "shallow cubes" (e.g., $c = 0.5$), indeed, all interpretations except the cube and the box-room. Because these 3-D interpretations are the ones we perceive then it seems likely that the brain assumes that the parallelogram texture elements in the *image* correspond to *squares* in the *world*. Writing this as the likelihood $p(x|c, \text{squares})$ will just confuse matters, so let's stick with the simpler $p(x|c)$ and assume that the surface texture consists of squares.

Given this new assumption, there are only two possible values for the three-dimensional shape: a convex cube, with convexity parameter value c_0, or a concave box-room, with convexity parameter value c_1. Crucially, both 3-D shapes are *equally* consistent with the image, so the image in figure 6.3b is perfectly ambiguous.

As an aside, if the squares at the image center were bigger than those elsewhere then this would indicate that the center squares were closer, and therefore that the 3-D object is a cube rather than a box-room. In this case, the likelihood value $p(x|c_0)$ would be greater than $p(x|c_1)$, and so we could choose the value of c associated with the greater likelihood value (i.e., c_0). The value c_0 associated with the maximum value of the likelihood is known as the "maximum likelihood estimate" (MLE). However, even if one of the likelihoods was greater, our decision would effectively ignore a valuable source of information regarding the most probable 3-D interpretation: previous experience.

How Probable Is That Shape?

Given the perfectly ambiguous stimulus in figure 6.3b, two values of the likelihood correspond to two possible values of the convexity parameter c, each of which implies a particular three-dimensional interpretation. Even though both these interpretations are equally consistent with the image, so that the likelihoods $p(x|c_0)$ and $p(x|c_1)$ are equal, they take no account of the prevalence of different 3-D shapes in the world. In other words, $p(x|c)$, the probability of the image x given a value for c, completely ignores the probability of being given any *particular* value of c by the world. So the likelihood $p(x|c)$ tells us the probability of the image data x for any particular value of c, but it takes no account of the fact that some values of c (i.e., the extent of 3-D convexity) occur more often than others.

Even though the data (i.e., the image) in figure 6.3b is equally consistent with two 3-D shapes, we tend to see one shape rather than the other. Equivalently, even though the data is equally consistent with c_0 and c_1, our perception suggests we favor c_0 over c_1. It is as if we somehow know that some 3-D shapes are intrinsically *more probable* in the world than other shapes, and therefore that some values of c are intrinsically more probable in the world than other values of c.

Supposing we take the likelihood value associated with each three-dimensional shape and to give it a *weighting* proportional to the prevalence of each 3-D shape in the world. For example, it may be that we encounter many more cubes than box-rooms; so the values of c given to us by the world are biased to favor c_0 over c_1. If our future is like our past (in terms of 3-D shapes) then we should expect to continue to encounter many more cubes than box-rooms. This suggests that we should have a bias for interpreting images as if they depict cubes rather than box-rooms. This, in turn, suggests that we should give a greater weighting to values of $p(x|c_0)$ than to values of $p(x|c_1)$. But how much greater should this weighting be? Well, if we have encountered twice as many cubes as box-rooms then it would seem sensible to give a weighting to $p(x|c_0)$ that is twice as great as the weighting given to $p(x|c_1)$.

If we express the number of cubes we have observed with convexity value c_0 as a proportion of all other shapes observed (i.e., all other observed

c values) then this is the probability of observing a cube shape, which can be written as $p(c_0)$. Similarly, the probability of observing a shape with convexity value c_1 can be written as $p(c_1)$. If we have observed twice as many cubes as box-rooms then the value of $p(c_0)$ is twice as great as that of $p(c_1)$. For example, we might find that $p(c_0) = 0.66$ and $p(c_1) = 0.33$. These probabilities are known as "prior probabilities," and one way to remember this is that they indicate the probability of encountering each value of the parameter c *before* we have observed the image $\mathbf{x}$.

If we weight the equal likelihood values $p(\mathbf{x}|c_0)$ and $p(\mathbf{x}|c_1)$ with their corresponding prior probabilities $p(c_0)$ and $p(c_1)$ then we obtain two new *unequal* conditional probabilities. Each of these is the probability of a specific value of c given the image data $\mathbf{x}$,

$$p(c_0|\mathbf{x}) = kp(\mathbf{x}|c_0)p(c_0)$$

$$p(c_1|\mathbf{x}) = kp(\mathbf{x}|c_1)p(c_1),$$

where k is a constant (whose value is not important here). Thus each of these represents the probability of a specified value of c *after* the probability of being given that value of c (by the world) has been taken into account. These are known as "posterior probabilities." (Strictly speaking, "prior" and "posterior" don't have to refer to temporal notions of "before" and "after," but this can be a useful way of getting to grips with these concepts.)

Let's put some numbers into these equations to see how it all works. We already know that the two likelihoods $p(\mathbf{x}|c_0)$ and $p(\mathbf{x}|c_1)$ are equal for figure 6.3b, so let's give them both a plausible value of 0.2. Given the values for the prior specified above, $p(c_0) = 0.66$ and $p(c_1) = 0.33$, this yields the posterior probabilities

$$p(c_0|\mathbf{x}) = 0.2 \times 0.66$$

$$\approx 0.13$$

$$p(c_1|\mathbf{x}) = 0.2 \times 0.33$$

$$\approx 0.07,$$

where the constant k has been omitted here. Thus, given the image data $\mathbf{x}$, the posterior probability that the shape parameter c is c_0 is twice as great as the posterior probability that the shape parameter is c_1. If we had to choose between these two parameter values then this implies that we should choose c_0. This is the value we should choose if we intend to take account of both the image data x *in addition to our past experience* (in the form of the prior $p(c)$) of different shapes in the world. This contrasts with a decision based on a comparison of the two likelihoods $p(\mathbf{x}|c_0)$ and $p(\mathbf{x}|c_1)$, which would be based on the image data alone and would take no account of previous experience in the form of the priors $p(c_0)$ and $p(c_1)$.

What we have just done, through a somewhat informal line of reasoning, is to apply the single most important equation in probability theory—Bayes' rule—to the problem of three-dimensional interpretation. Indeed, the whole process of finding the most probable value of the convexity parameter c is an example of Bayesian inference.

The observant reader will have noticed that the sum of posterior probabilities in the example above is about 0.2, and not unity (1.0), which seems almost like declaring that a coin can land heads up with probability 0.13 and heads down with probability 0.07. Because a coin must land either heads up or heads down, the total probability that it lands *either* heads up *or* heads down is of course unity, and not 0.2. If there are only two possible values for a parameter, each of which has a posterior probability, then it follows that the sum of these probabilities must also be unity, a defining feature of a *probability distribution*. As it turns out, the sum above is *not* unity because we have omitted the constant term k. The value of this constant can be shown to be $k = 1/p(\mathbf{x})$, where $p(\mathbf{x})$ is the overall probability of observing the image data $\mathbf{x}$. But the reason we have omitted this constant term is because knowing its value makes *no difference* to which posterior probability has the greatest value, and therefore doesn't affect which value of c we choose. For example, if we knew that $p(\mathbf{x}) = 0.2$ then both equations would get multiplied by $k = 5$, and the correct posterior probabilities would then sum to unity: $p(c_0|\mathbf{x}) = 0.65$ and $p(c_1|\mathbf{x}) = 0.35$; $0.65 + 0.35 = 1.0$. However, because both equations would get multiplied by the *same* number (5), the *relative* magnitudes of the posterior probabilities would remain unaltered, so we would still choose c_0 rather than c_1. Thus the value of $p(\mathbf{x})$ has no impact on the chosen value of c, which is why we do not care about its value.

The general form of the equation used to perform Bayesian inference is called "Bayes' rule" or "Bayes' theorem":

$$p(c \mid \mathbf{x}) = \frac{p(\mathbf{x} \mid c)p(c)}{p(\mathbf{x})},$$

which is easier to remember as

posterior = $k \times$ likelihood $\times$ prior.

Bayes' rule gives us an excellent way to combine evidence based on current sensory inputs (e.g., an image) with previous experience (or even innate knowledge) to arrive at a statistically optimal estimate of what in the world gave rise to any particular image.

Generalizing Bayes' Rule

We can make more general use of Bayes' rule if we back up a little and again consider all possible values of the convexity parameter c. If we plot a graph of how probable the image x is given each value of c then we obtain a *likelihood function*, as shown in figure 6.4a. This shows how the probability of observing the data x changes as the value of the convexity parameter c is varied continuously.

It may at first appear nonsensical to speak of how probable the image x is given each value of c. However, if we consider the set of images from all objects with a given convexity value then we would find, for example, that the image x before us is most commonly observed for some pair of values c_0' and c_1' that correspond to the locations of the peaks in figure 6.4a (not equal to c_0 and c_1). As before, for a convexity value of c_0, the value of the likelihood $p(x|c_0)$ is 0.2, and for a convexity value of c_1, the value of the likelihood $p(x|c_0)$ is also 0.2. Be careful not to be confused by the fact that the image of the box-room shown in figure 6.4d is the same as the image of the cube shown in figure 6.4e (because we already know that both 3-D shapes yield the same image).

Notice that the square texture elements on the surface of the box-room (c_1) yield, not squares, but quadrilaterals in the image shown in figure 6.4d. However, as the 3-D shape defined by different values of c is made more "flat," the squares on its surface yield image texture elements that are increasingly square, so that, if the three-dimensional shape were flat $(c = 0)$, then each square texture element on its surface would yield a *square* in the image.

Recall that the likelihood is the probability of observing a specific image given a putative value (e.g., c_0 or c_1) of the convexity c parameter that defines the 3-D shape of the object. Consequently, the probability of observing the image of a box-room (figure 6.4d) shrinks as we consider values of c *greater than* c_1. A similar argument implies that the probability of observing the image of a box-room also shrinks as we consider values of c *less than* c_1. This reduction in the value of the likelihood $p(x|c)$ on either side of c_1 is reflected in figure 6.4a, which falls away on either side of c_1. Of course, all of this also applies to the image of a cube, so the likelihood values also fall away either side of c_0 (figure 6.4e).

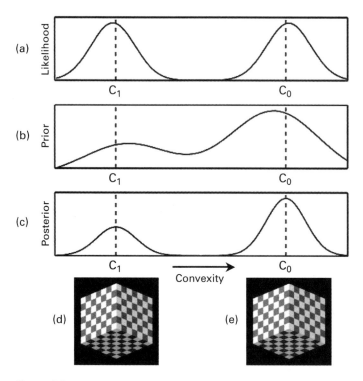

Figure 6.4

Three key ingredients of the Bayesian framework. The shape of the object in figure 6.3b could be either a convex cube with convexity value c_0 or a concave box-room with convexity value c_1. (a) Likelihood function $p(\mathbf{x}|c)$. The probability of the retinal image $\mathbf{x}$ in figure 6.3 varies as shapes with different values of the shape parameter c are considered. This likelihood function has two equal peaks that correspond to convex and concave 3-D shapes. (b) Prior $p(c)$. The frequency with which shapes having each value of convexity are observed is reflected in the structure of the prior probability density function. This implies that shapes that are convex with convexity value c_0 are encountered more often than shapes that are concave with convexity value c_1. The posterior $p(c|\mathbf{x})$ is the product of corresponding heights in (a) and (b). Its graph shows the probability that different values of convexity c gave rise to the image $\mathbf{x}$ in figure 6.3. This posterior probability density function has two unequal peaks, with the larger peak corresponding to an estimate the true convexity c_0 (an almost perfectly accurate estimate in this example).

We can now see why the likelihood function has two peaks, one close to c_0 and one close to c_1. We can also see why the heights of these two peaks are the same (because both of the corresponding three-dimensional shapes are *equally* consistent with the image x). As in the previous section, the equal heights of these two peaks in the likelihood function mean that it can't be used to choose which of the two possible values of c, and therefore which 3-D interpretation, is more probable.

The likelihood function implies that, if we were given the values c_0 and c_1 then we would find that both values would yield the image x with the same probability. However, *the probabilities of being given the shapes c_0 and c_1 by the world in the first place are not the same.* In fact, we can plot a graph of the *prior probability density function*, denoted as $p(c)$, which shows the probability of encountering 3-D shapes with each value of c, like the graph in figure 6.4b.

When we considered individual values of c in the previous section, we obtained individual values of the posterior probability $p(c|x)$ by weighting each likelihood by its prior probability. We can follow the same logic here with the continuous range of convexity values in figure 6.4a–c. We proceed by weighting each value of the likelihood function in figure 6.4a by the corresponding value of the prior probability density function in figure 6.4b, in order to obtain a *posterior probability density function*, denoted as $p(c|x)$, in figure 6.4c. This weighting amounts to multiplying each height on the likelihood function $p(x|c)$ in figure 6.4a by the corresponding height of the prior probability density function $p(c)$ in figure 6.4b to obtain the posterior probability density function $p(c|x)$ in figure 6.4c. When the context is unambiguous, we'll refer to the posterior probability density, likelihood, and prior probability density functions simply as the "posterior," "likelihood," and "prior." Also, note that the quantity $p(c|x)$ is a *number* when we consider a specific value of c (e.g., if $c = c_0$ then $p(c_0|x) = 0.13$), but when considered over all possible values of c it defines a probability density function, represented by the curve in figure 6.4c, for example.

The posterior, which takes account of the prevalence of different parameter values in the world, can be used to find the value of c that most probably gave rise to the image x. Specifically, the value of c associated with the peak in the posterior of figure 6.4c, known as the "maximum a posteriori" (MAP) estimate, is the best estimate of the true convexity c_0. As before, this contrasts with a decision based the likelihood function that would be based on the image data alone, which would take no account of previous experience in the form of the prior. In this instance, the difference between the best estimate based on the likelihood (the maximum likelihood estimate, MLE) and the best estimate based on the posterior (the MAP) is quite small, but it can be substantial. More importantly, on average, the MAP is guaranteed to be more accurate than the MLE.

Finally, note that the prior and the posterior are both *probability density functions* (pdfs), which means that their individual values sum to unity. For example, the sum of values of the posterior $p(c|x)$ is unity, when considered over all possible values of c (not x). However, the likelihood function $p(x|c)$ is unusual, inasmuch as it defines the probability of the data x given c, *not* when considered over all possible values of x, but over all values of c; consequently, its values do not sum to unity, and therefore it's *not* a probability density function.

Bayes' Rule Increases Accuracy, on Average

Even though the estimate of the convexity parameter c given by the posterior (the MAP) is, on average, *more* accurate than the estimate given by the likelihood function (the MLE), it can occasionally be *less* accurate. For example, in figure 6.4a, the location of each peak in the likelihood function identifies a value of c that is most consistent with the image x, provided information regarding prior experience is ignored. We have seen that the structure of the prior ensures that the posterior also has two peaks, but one of these is higher than the other, and the location of this peak specifies the value of the MAP estimate of c_0. In this example, the MAP estimate is exactly equal to the true value c_0. More generally, the influence of the prior on the posterior not only allows a MAP estimate to be obtained, but this estimate is usually different from the true value c_0. Here's why.

Unlike the example shown in figure 6.4c, neither of the peaks in the posterior usually coincides exactly with c_0 or c_1. Recall that, in this example, the prior simply reflects the relative preponderance of three-dimensional convexity values in the world, so there's no reason why peaks in the prior should coincide with peaks in the likelihood function for a given image x. When the prior is multiplied, point for point, by the likelihood function, the peaks in the likelihood get "moved" (by the influence of the prior) to peaks in the posterior that are closer to peaks in the prior. When averaged over all possible 3-D shapes (i.e., values of c), the estimates of convexity c based on the posterior are, on average, more accurate than estimates based on the likelihood. However, it is important to note that this does not hold true for "any old prior," but it is true *if the* prior used is an *accurate repre-*

sentation of the *prevalence of different values* of c in the world, which we will call the "world prior" here.

Thus, if the brain uses Bayes' rule then its estimate of three-dimensional shape is, on average, accurate, *provided* it makes use of the world prior. In other words, interpretations of retinal images that rely on previous experience are, on average, better than those which ignore previous experience. This suggests that the brain could, in effect, be acting as a *Bayesian inference engine*, a kind of *perfect guessing machine*. Even though these guesses aren't always correct, provided they are based on Bayes' rule, it can be shown that no other (i.e., non-Bayesian) method can do any better.

A Prior for Face Convexity?

This general formulation of Bayes' rule can be applied to almost any problem in vision. For example, the amount of depth perceived in the image of figure 6.5a depends on at least three entities: the image data, the prior for face shape, and the prior for lighting direction. We have already seen in chapter 1 how the assumption of face convexity can force the lighting direction assumed by the brain to "flip" from above to below. As a less dramatic but no less important consideration, just *how* convex the brain assumes the face to be can influence exactly *where* it assumes the light source to be. For example, for the brain to perceive the image in figure

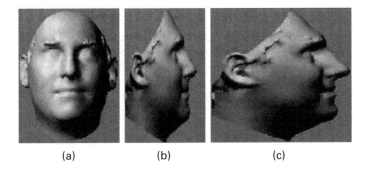

(a)   (b)   (c)

Figure 6.5
The inherent ambiguity of image shading. (a) Normal human face. (b) Compressed human face. (c) Stretched human face. Both the compressed face in (b) and the stretched face in (c) yield exactly the same retinal image as the normal face in (a), when viewed from the front. This implies that the depth we see when we look at the image in (a) is determined partly by our own perceptual bias, and partly by the image. Adapted with permission from Kersten & Yuille 2003.

6.5a to have the depth profile depicted in figure 6.5b, it must assume that the light source is almost directly in front of the face. In contrast, for it to perceive the image in figure 6.5a to have the depth profile depicted in figure 6.5c, the brain must assume the light source is almost directly above the face.

To keep things simple, let's fix the assumed lighting direction at an intermediate angle, consistent with the depth profile depicted in figure 6.6e. Of course, even if we do so, the prior for face convexity can still influence the perceived depth profile, but there will be more to say on that topic later.

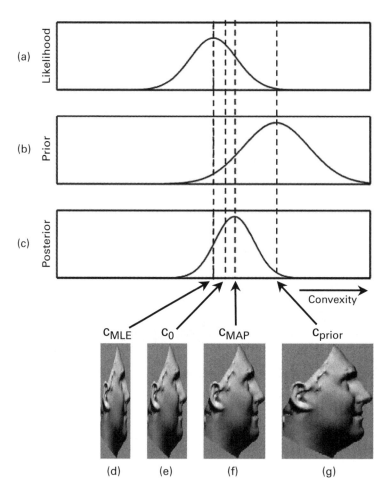

Figure 6.6
Interpreting the 3-D depth profile for the face shown in figure 6.5a. These distributions are for illustration purposes only.

If we assume the lighting source is in a fixed direction then the probability of the image data $\mathbf{x}$ given a particular convexity value c is written as $p(\mathbf{x}|c)$. We should really write this as $p(\mathbf{x}|c, \theta_0)$, where θ_0 represents the fixed lighting direction, but we will use $p(\mathbf{x}|c)$ for simplicity. As in the previous example, the true value of the face convexity is c_0, which corresponds to the profile shown in figure 6.6e. If we plot a graph of $p(\mathbf{x}|c)$ for all values of c, then we obtain the likelihood function shown in figure 6.6a. If we use this likelihood function of c to choose an estimate of face convexity then we would select the value c_{MLE} associated with the peak, as shown in figure 6.6a and d. Because c_{MLE} corresponds to the maximum value of likelihood function, it is the maximum likelihood estimate of the true value c_0.

However, our everyday experience informs us that faces have a restricted range of convexity values. This effectively defines a prior distribution $p(c)$ over all possible values of the face convexity parameter c, as shown in figure 6.6b. For example, if you were raised on the planet Flatface then your prior would be to the left of the prior shown in figure 6.6b, and you would perceive figure 6.5a as if it had the "squashed" profile in figure 6.5b. Conversely, if you were raised on planet Bignose then your prior would be to the right of the prior shown in figure 6.6b, and you would perceive the image in figure 6.5a as if it depicted the elongated profile depicted in figure 6.5c.

The prior shown in figure 6.6b is centered on a specific value of convexity c_{prior}, which corresponds to the face shown in figure 6.6g. The probability of different convexity values is given by the height of the prior for each value of convexity c. For example, this prior implies that face convexity values at the true value c_0 shown in figure 6.6e are not very probable. In other words, according to this prior, faces with the profile shown in figure 6.6e are only rarely observed, so that such faces are, by definition, improbable. In contrast, faces with the profile shown in figure 6.6g are, according to this prior, most common.

The posterior $p(c|\mathbf{x})$, obtained by multiplying the heights of corresponding points on the likelihood and prior, is shown in figure 6.6c. As before, the location c_{MAP} of the peak in the posterior defines the MAP estimate of the true convexity value c_0. Note that, in this example, c_{MAP} does not correspond to the true convexity c_0, nor does it correspond to the peak of the prior located at c_{prior}. Instead, the location c_{MAP} of the peak in the posterior lies between c_{MLE} and c_{prior}. The proximity of c_{MAP} to c_0 and c_{prior} depends on the relative widths of their corresponding distributions, as described below. This is as it should be if the prior acts as a moderating influence on the likelihood, where this moderation depends both on the reliability of the image data and on the form of the prior. If this Bayesian inference takes place in your brain then your posterior $p(c|\mathbf{x})$ has a peak that is biased by your own personal experience of faces. As explained in the previous section, when considered over all faces, following Bayes' rule guarantees that such estimates are as accurate as possible.

Noisy Images

As we have seen above, a peak in the likelihood function is not necessarily associated with the true value of convexity c_0. This, it was argued, is because other three-dimensional objects with the convexity value c_0 are more common than a cube (or a face) with convexity value c_0. A more conventional account of why the likelihood function does not usually yield the true value c_0 of convexity can be obtained by disregarding all other 3-D shapes, and instead considering variations in the image of a specific 3-D shape (such as a cube or a face) caused by the effects of noise. Such an account serves as a bridge between the noise-free account given above and those given in standard texts on Bayesian analysis.

The luminance levels at different points on the retina are measured by photoreceptors, which are, like all measurement devices, imperfect, as shown in figure 6.7. The output of each photoreceptor depends on the luminance within a small patch of the retinal image but changes from moment to moment due to stray photons and to its own spontaneous fluctuations. As light levels fall, so the balance in the output of each photoreceptor tips in favor of noise. Furthermore, retinal ganglion cells, which collate the noisy outputs of photoreceptors, contribute additional random changes to their outputs. Together, these random fluctuations ensure that the information received by the brain contains random errors, which increase under low-light conditions. The net effect is that the brain sometimes receives information consistent with a noisy image $\mathbf{x}'$ (read as "x prime") when the noise-free image $\mathbf{x}$ is actually on the retina. Because the noise changes from moment to moment, let's write the resultant temporal sequence of images as $\mathbf{x}'_1, \mathbf{x}'_2, \mathbf{x}'_3, \ldots$, using the term $\mathbf{x}'$ to refer to an arbitrary noisy image.

Now, as far as the brain is concerned, the image on the retina is not $\mathbf{x}$ but a noisy version $\mathbf{x}'$ that changes from moment to moment. Accordingly, the likelihood function, which is based only on the available data, depends on the current noisy image $\mathbf{x}'$ and therefore also changes from moment to moment. So the likelihood function plotted in figure 6.6a is really a snapshot taken at one moment in time. Accordingly, this likelihood function

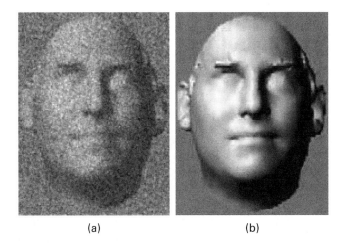

(a)   (b)

Figure 6.7
Schematic image x'. (a) Photoreceptor outputs represented in response to the image
x. (b) Outputs after they've been corrupted by random noise (e.g., under low-light
conditions). The gray level of each pixel on the page in (a) represents the output of
a single photoreceptor.

should be written as $p(x'|c)$ rather than $p(x|c)$ because its height at each
point refers to the probability of the noisy (i.e., measured) image x' for a
given value of c, rather than the probability of the noise-free image x for
a given value of c. Just as the data x' changes due to noise, so the MLE also
changes, which implies that the MLE is usually in error.

Adopting the same Bayesian line of reasoning as above, this error can
be reduced by making use of prior experience to provide an estimate of
the true value of convexity based on the posterior, an estimate that is, on
average, better than that the one provided by the likelihood function. In
other words, bringing previous experience to bear when estimating the
shapes of faces increases the accuracy of those estimates.

Evidence versus Experience

If the depth cues given by an image are weak, as in figure 6.3a then the
posterior, and therefore the perceived depth, depends almost exclusively
on the form of the prior. For example, if we had not fixed the lighting
direction then the image in figure 6.5a (repeated in figure 6.7b) would be
equally consistent with all values of convexity, so that the likelihood function would be a horizontal line. In this case, the posterior would be exactly

the same as the prior, and therefore c_{MAP} would correspond to the peak of the prior. In other words, the convexity you see when you look at the image in figure 6.5a would be determined only by your previous experience of faces. This example lies at one extreme of a continuum in which the relative importance of evidence (image data) versus previous experience varies.

At the other extreme, if the 3-D face in figure 6.7b were viewed under bright illumination with two eyes then shape-from-stereopsis cues would massively restrict the possible 3-D shapes that could account for the image data. Without going into details, this would make the broad bump in the likelihood function shown in figure 6.6a collapse to a narrow spike (known as a "delta function"). Its narrowness would ensure that this spike would appear almost unscathed in the posterior, and at the same location as the spike in the likelihood function (i.e., the MLE = MAP). In other words, if the image data is essentially free of noise and in all other respects unambiguous then the impact of the prior on the location of the peak (MAP) in the posterior is negligible.

Thus, in a world where evidence in the form of image data has an unambiguous (e.g., 3-D) interpretation and is free of noise, there would be little need for priors, and therefore little need of Bayes' rule. However, it is not difficult to experience visual noise by walking out into the dusk in order to see many shapes that are not there, to view a noise-free but evidence-poor image in order to see a specific face convexity where no particular degree of convexity is implied by the image (figure 6.7b), or to see a luminance edge where there is none (figure 1.1).

Bayesian Wars

Whereas engineers and physicists view Bayes' rule as plain common sense, many statisticians and psychologists view it with deep suspicion. Indeed, the ongoing skirmishes and battles that surround the debate over the status and application of Bayes' rule (Jones & Love 2011) can, on occasion, escalate into Bayesian wars.

Edwin T. Jaynes, who was one of the key players in the development of modern Bayesian theory, pointed out that much of the heat of this debate depends on ideological arguments regarding the interpretation of probability, and that there is actually little to debate if the mathematical infrastructure and scientific utility of different methods are compared (Jaynes & Bretthorst 2003). Specifically, in setting up rules for calculating with probabilities, we would insist that the result of such calculations should tally with our everyday experience of the physical world, just as surely as we would insist that $1 + 1 = 2$. Indeed, as Richard T. Cox (1946) showed, insisting that probabilities be combined with each other in accordance with certain common sense principles leads to a unique set of rules, a set that includes Bayes' rule.

Bayes' rule has been used to combine evidence from different sources in a wide variety of different contexts, such as computer vision, signal processing, medical diagnosis, and legal proceedings, where it has been criticized as "a recipe for confusion and misjudgment, possibly even among counsel, but very probably among judges and, as we conclude, almost certainly among jurors" (Haigh 2003, p. 609). In light of such a dogmatic, yet unsurprising declarations should make us determined to be absolutely clear about the logical status of Bayes' rule. Bayes' rule is not like a "rule of thumb" which was discovered in the process of observing how probabilities happen to interact, or by observing the fall of a die, for example. It is not a hypothesis awaiting empirical tests of its validity, like "red sky at night, shepherd's delight." Bayes' rule is more properly called a mathematical *theorem*, where "theorem" is the mathematicians' word for "statement." Like most theorems, it can be proved true or false, and Bayes' theorem is true. Consequently, *there cannot be any debate regarding the truth of Bayes' theorem.* So why does it generate so much emotion?

Within the realms of perceptual research, this debate is fueled partly by misunderstandings regarding its logical status (i.e., whether or not it is true), and partly by the suspicion that the prior represents some form of mathematical sleight of hand, despite valiant attempts at explaining Bayes' rule within the context of psychology (Dienes 2008; Scholl 2005), and in popular science (McGrayne 2011). For example, a common objection is that the context of a stimulus affects how it is perceived, and that this suffices to explain certain illusions. However, the word "context" here is being used to carry a heavy load, a load that it cannot possibly bear.

Consider the choice represented by two explanations for an illusion, like the one shown in figure 1.8. One relies heavily on the context (e.g., the context being upright or inverted), and the other explains it in terms of a prior distribution, which specifies precisely how probable each possible lighting direction is (when considered all "around the clock"). Both are indeed explanations, but the use of a prior allows us to predict exactly what will be perceived for any given stimulus orientation. In other words, the use of priors and the Bayesian framework, when properly applied, promises to take us out of the purely linguistic realms of description regarding the role of context. What little debate there is to be had within perceptual psychology involves whether the brain follows Bayes' theorem, with all of the attendant implications regarding how priors are learned and updated (Berniker, Voss, & Kording 2010) or inherited (Stone 2011).

Whereas a Bayesian analysis of data from experiments on perception is usually possible, such an analysis often relies on the *assumption* that perception is Bayesian in character, but says nothing about whether it involves Bayesian inference. In contrast, experiments designed to test whether perceptual processes rely on Bayesian inference can shed light on this debate. To date, almost every experiment (Girschick, Landy, & Simoncelli 2011; Knill & Saunders 2003; Knill 2007b) that has applied such a test suggests that the brain appears, to all intents and purposes, to behave *as if* it is a Bayesian inference engine.

In summary, Bayes' theorem is not just a convenient rule that happens to work. It's part of a set of rules that are logically implied by our insistence that such rules yield results that conform to the behavior of the physical world. More important, it's a rule that the brain seems to follow as a general principle for interpreting data from the senses (Friston 2009).

Brains and Bayesian Inference

It is only natural to ask how and where Bayesian inference might be implemented in the brain. As to *how* it might, there's a large literature that explores the computational capabilities of neuronal function in the context of Bayesian inference (Deneve, Latham, & Pouget 2001; Ganguli & Simoncelli 2010; Girschick, Landy, & Simoncelli 2011; Knill & Pouget 2004; Kover & Bao 2010). This literature suggests that, although the case remains unproven, there's no reason to doubt that neurons have both the computational power and the means to perform Bayesian inference if required to do so.

Additionally, regarding the question of *how*, the following represents one possible implementation. Consider a neuron that responds preferentially to the image of a line on the retina at a specific angle (e.g., a simple cell; see chapter 3). When the image of a line falls on the retina, the neuron has an output which represents the degree of mismatch between its preferred orientation and the orientation of the line on the retina. In other words, the neuron's output may be said to represent the probability of the image line (i.e., data x) given the preferred orientation of the neuron. If we use c_i to represent the preferred orientation here then the neuron's output can be considered to be a measure of the likelihood $p(x|c_i)$. If the synaptic strength that connects this "likelihood" neuron to a "posterior" neuron is proportional to the prior $p(c_i)$ then the output of the "posterior" neuron is a measure of the posterior probability $p(c_i|\mathbf{x}) = p(\mathbf{x}|c_i)p(c_i)$ (we have ignored the constant k here). Even though there is no reason to suppose that Bayes' rule is implemented in this way, this example serves to demonstrate one of many possible ways that Bayes' rule *could* be implemented by the brain.

Regarding the question of *where*, the answer should be "pretty much everywhere in the brain," although there is as yet little empirical evidence to support this claim. We will not pursue these matters further here, mainly because they are secondary to findings that suggest, irrespective of where and how it is achieved, the brain does indeed seem to perform Bayesian inference.

Marr and Bayes

The Bayesian framework could be said to represent the apotheosis of Marr's computational approach to vision. In common with the computational level within Marr's framework, a Bayesian analysis explicitly takes almost no account of the particular machinery that performs the computational legwork required in order to solve a given problem in vision, like depth perception. In particular, the notion of priors corresponds to Marr's use of certain constraints to help solve a particular vision problem. More generally, the Bayesian framework allows the computational nature of a problem to be made explicit, unhindered by a consideration of how or where specific parameters are represented and manipulated by the brain. Of course, it can be argued that such unfettered theorizing rapidly loses contact with anything to do with how the brain works in practice. However, as always in science, experimental evidence is the final arbiter regarding the validity of any theory, even Bayesian ones.

Conclusion

It may seem odd to rely on a mathematical equation to explain how vision at all levels of analysis, from photoreceptors to three-dimensional perceptions, can be rescued from the effects of missing information. But the fact remains that some information is always missing, due either to noise or to an impoverished or ambiguous image, and Bayes' rule provides a rational basis for how to use previous experience as a proxy for this missing information.

Even though Bayes' paper was published in 1763, its role in perception has been explored only in the last fifteen years (e.g., Beierholm, Quartz, & Shams 2009; Brainard et al. 2006; Doya et al. 2007; Fischer & Pena 2011; Girshick, Landy, & Simoncelli 2011; Kersten, Mamassian, & Yuille 2004; Knill 2007a, 2007b; Knill & Richards 1996; Kording & Wolpert 2004; Purves & Lotto 2003; Salinas 2011; Stocker & Simoncelli 2006; Stone, Kerrigan, & Porrill 2009). And whereas only a fool would deny that perception depends both on the retinal image and on past experience or generic assumptions about the statistical structure of the physical world, only an idiot would claim that the particular manner in which these two are combined *must* be Bayesian in nature. Having said that, in almost every instance that has been subjected to experimental verification (e.g., Knill & Saunders 2003), so far, the idiot would have been proved right.

7   The Color of Information

It appears likely that a major function of the perceptual machinery is to strip away some of the redundancy of stimulation, to describe or encode incoming information in a form more economical than that in which it impinges on the receptors.
—Fred Attneave (1954)

Impressions

Who is number one? You are number six. What do you want? Information. You won't get it. Given that you had two alternatives, to agree or disagree to provide information, your negative response has just given us exactly one bit of information, thank you. Well, you won't be getting any more. Given that you had two alternatives, to tell us you will or you won't provide more information, your response gives us another bit, thank you again. That's a low-down, two-bit trick to play. We already knew that, so your response has given us no information. I am glad to hear it. Given that you had two alternatives, to be glad or not to be glad, your response gives us another bit; please continue. I can see that the only way for me not to provide information is to be silent. Fair enough. Was that your final bit? It was. Apparently not . . .

There is something odd about color vision. First, the three types of color cones in the human eye respond to colored light in a way you would not obviously choose if you were designing a camera. The cone types supposedly sensitive to "red" and "green" light respond to colors are so similar that each makes the other seem redundant. Second, the cones that respond to blue light are relatively insensitive. Third, the proportion of blue cones is vanishingly small. Fourth, traditionally, there are thought to be three primary colors (red, green, and blue), and these correspond to the three cone types in the retina. However, when considered in terms of color *aftereffects*, there seem to be four "primary colors," such that staring at red

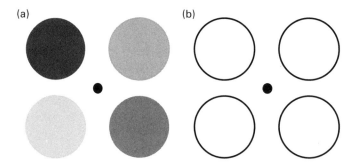

Figure 7.1 (plate 12)
Color aftereffect. (a) Four disks colored red, green, yellow, and blue. (b) Same four disks without color. Fix your gaze on the central black dot in (a) for about 30 seconds, then transfer your gaze to the black dot in (b) and notice the perceived color of the disks. Why does red give a green and blue a yellow aftereffect? From Frisby & Stone 2010.

yields a green aftereffect (and vice versa), while staring at blue yields a yellow aftereffect (and vice versa), as shown in figure 7.1 (plate 12).

We will explore some of these quirks by taking an unconventional approach to color vision. The central concept that motivates this chapter draws on a number of related ideas, most notably, redundancy reduction (Atick & Redlich 1992), predictive coding (Rao & Ballard 1999; Srinavasen, Laughlin, & Dubs 1982), maximizing sparseness (Foldiak & Young 1995), minimizing energy (Niven, Anderson, & Laughlin 2007), independent component analysis (Bell & Sejnowski 1995; Stone 2004), and efficient coding (Atick, Li, & Redlich 1992; Attneave 1954; Barlow 1961; Laughlin 1981). These ideas have developed from original work by Claude Shannon and Warren Weaver on information theory, which sparked a huge amount of research into information processing in the nervous system in the 1950s and 1960s. Within the realms of perception, both Fred Attneave (1954) and Horace Barlow (1961) have contributed much. In particular, Barlow's work has been instrumental in the development of the efficient coding hypothesis.

A recent resurgence of interest in information theory in the context of perception has led to a rapid development of ideas, facilitated both by the existence of modern camera systems capable of measuring the spectral properties of natural scenes and by developments in neurophysiological recording techniques. The general information-theoretic approach has been applied to color, but also to the recoding of image information by retinal ganglion cells (see "Logan's Need to Know" in chapter 3), and to the efficient coding of different image properties such as luminance, line orientation, and stereopsis (Zhaoping forthcoming).

Rather than describing the human color system and then wondering why it evolved to be that way, we will instead consider what sort of color vision system an engineer might design, and then compare that with what we find in the human visual system. If we do this properly then we should experience a reversal in our line of reasoning by the end of this chapter. Rather than asking: why is the visual system built the way it is?, we'll end up asking this: given the nature of the problems the visual system has to solve, why would it be built any differently from the way that it is?

Color and Light

Light, Cones, and Rods
Visible light is part of the spectrum of electromagnetic radiation, as shown in figure 7.2 (plate 13). Because light behaves like a wave, it can be defined in terms of its wavelength, which is the distance between consecutive wave peaks (figure 7.3, plate 14). At one end of the spectrum, electromagnetic radiation has extremely short wavelengths, like the gamma (γ) radiation

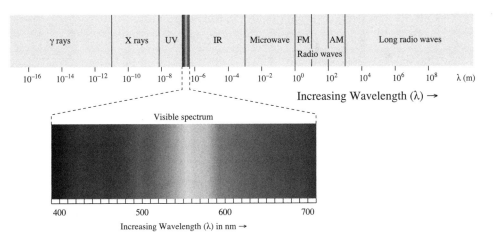

Figure 7.2 (plate 13)
Spectrum of electromagnetic radiation, showing an expanded version of the spectrum's visible part between 400 and 700 nm (where 1,000 nm is a thousandth of a millimeter). Light behaves like a wave, and the distance between consecutive peaks is its wavelength, represented by the Greek letter lambda (λ). Figure by Philip Ronan. Courtesy Creative Commons.

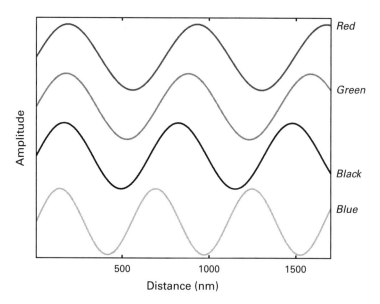

Figure 7.3 (plate 14)

Comparison of wavelengths for retinal photoreceptors. The red curve shows the wavelength (564 nm) of light to which red L-cones are most sensitive, green shows the wavelength (533 nm) to which green M-cones are most sensitive, and blue shows the wavelength (420 nm) to which blue S-cones are most sensitive. The black curve shows the wavelength (498 nm) to which rods are most sensitive.

released in nuclear bombs, which has a wavelength of 0.001 nanometer (nm; a nanometer is a millionth of a millimeter). At the other end of the spectrum, electromagnetic radiation has extremely long wavelengths, like the radio waves in the 100- to 1,000-meter range used by AM radio stations. Visible light appears to us as the colors of the rainbow: red, orange, yellow, green, blue, indigo, and violet (which can be memorized as the name ROY G BIV).

It is worth noting that light itself is *not* colored. Color is what we see when light rays with a particular range of wavelengths strike the retina. Isaac Newton (1704, p. 125) was probably the first to make this subtle but critical distinction when he wrote that "the Rays to speak properly are not coloured. In them there is nothing else than a certain Power and Disposition to stir up a Sensation of this or that Colour."

As mentioned in chapter 2, there are three types of color cones, which are sensitive to light that appears red, green, and blue to us. The amount of light absorbed at each wavelength by each cone type defines its *tuning*

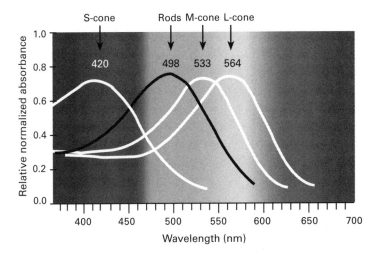

Figure 7.4 (plate 15)

Photoreceptor sensitivity to different wavelengths of light. The sensitivity of each photoreceptor type to different wavelengths of light defines its relative spectral absorbance, or *tuning curve*. Each curve is the tuning curve of one photoreceptor type. There are three cone types: L (red), M (green) and S (blue). The number above each curve gives the peak sensitivity wavelength in nanometers (nm). Based on data from Bowmaker & Dartnall 1980; reproduced from Frisby & Stone 2010.

curve, as shown in figure 7.4 (plate 15). Cones sensitive to long-wavelength light that appears red are conventionally labeled "L-cones," cones sensitive to medium-wavelength light that appears green are labeled "M-cones," and cones sensitive to short-wavelength light that appears blue are labeled "S-cones." However, for simplicity, let's refer to these as "red," "green," and "blue cones," respectively, with the understanding that we mean only the perceived color of light to which each cone is most sensitive, as shown in figure 7.3. The fact there are exactly three types of color cones explains why almost any color we are capable of seeing can be constructed using three colors of light. This is why a TV picture can be constructed using triplets of red-, green-, and blue-colored pixels, as in (figure 7.5, plate 16).

Cones mediate daylight vision, but are not sensitive enough to be useful under low-light conditions. The rods are much more sensitive than cones, and are essentially bleached out by daylight. However, under low-light conditions after about 30 minutes, they rebuild their stores of photosensitive pigment called "rhodopsin" to mediate night vision. Because there's only one type of rod, the brain has no way to use the outputs of rods to

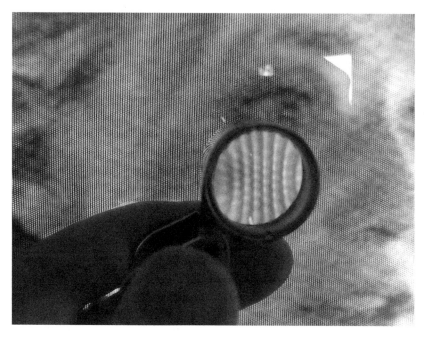

Figure 7.5 (plate 16)
A color television picture consists of a mosaic of triplets of red-, green-, and blue-colored pixels, which can be seen through a magnifying glass. The blue pixels are quite dark here because the underlying picture is of a face, which contains very little blue.

discriminate different colors, which is why we do not see colors under low-light conditions.

There's a Hole in the Sky Where the Light Gets In

Why has evolution given us eyes that are sensitive to wavelengths between 400 and 700 nm and not to others beyond that range? There are three related reasons.

First, the energy in sunlight peaks within the visible range of wavelengths between 400 and 700 nm; it falls off sharply for shorter wavelengths, and more gradually for longer wavelengths, as shown in figure 7.6 (plate 17). Second, the Earth's atmosphere blocks wavelengths shorter than about 400 nm and attenuates those longer than 700 nm, due to the scattering of light by air molecules and to absorbance by water molecules in the atmosphere. And third, seawater, in which all eyes first evolved, is most transparent to wavelengths at about 500 nm, effectively blocking wave-

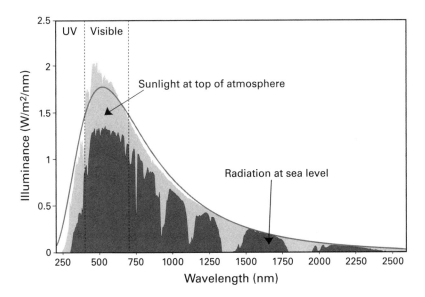

Figure 7.6 (plate 17)
Most terrestrial animals see light with wavelengths between 400 and 700 nm because that's where sunlight's energy peaks. The yellow shading shows which wavelengths dominate at the top of the atmosphere, whereas red shows how much light energy at each wavelength survives sea level. The vertical axis indicates watts (energy per second) per square meter at each wavelength. By RA Rohde, Global Warming Art project, Creative Commons.

lengths shorter than about 200 nm and becoming increasingly opaque to those longer than 500 nm. In essence, our eyes and those of most other terrestrial animals have evolved to see the range of wavelengths that dominate the natural spectrum of light after it has passed through the atmosphere.

Information, Bit by Bit

Big Message, Small Wires
There is an information bottleneck at the back of the eye, where the information from 126 million photoreceptors gets squeezed into one million nerve fibers of the optic nerve. Because the red and green cone types have such similar tuning curves (figure 7.4, plate 15), light that evokes a response from a red cone, also induces a response from a nearby green cone, and, these responses are usually similar in magnitude. If these red and green cones had their own private nerve fibers to send their outputs

along then, clearly, the messages traveling down these two nerve fibers would be similar. Given the information bottleneck, this would obviously be a wasteful use of the capacity of these channels of communication. But there's a way to send information along channels (be they wires, nerve fibers or lengths of string), without wasting channel capacity. Before describing how this can be done we first need to define what is meant by "information."

Navigating Information Theory, Bit by Bit

The theory of information, first published by Claude Shannon in 1948, provides the tools to measure pure information, unfettered by the demands of physics or biology (Shannon 1948; Shannon & Weaver 1949). In essence, the theory states that each *information channel* has a finite *capacity*, some of which is usually wasted, and that the full capacity of information channels can be achieved by judicious *recoding* of the messages to be communicated.

The unit of information is the *bit* (from "*b*inary" and "dig*it*"; a zero or a one). One bit of information tells you which alternative to choose between two *equally likely* alternatives. Imagine you are standing at a fork in the road (of life, for example), at point A in figure 7.7. If you have no

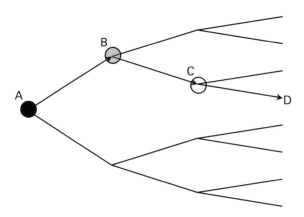

Figure 7.7
How many roads must a man walk down? Each fork in a road requires one bit* of information for you to choose the right road to take. After one fork at A, you've eliminated half of the eight possible roads, leaving four. After the second fork at B, you've eliminated half of the four remaining possible roads, leaving only two. After the third fork at C, you've eliminated half of the two remaining possible roads, leaving only one destination. Thus three bits of information allow you to navigate through three forks in the road, and to choose one out of eight possible destinations.

prior information about which road to choose then the fork represents two equally likely alternatives. If I tell you which of these roads to choose (left) then you have received one bit of information (a crucial bit, in this case). If we define "left" as 1 and "right" as 0 then I can convey that bit of information to you with a binary digit.

Now imagine that you stroll on down that road and come to another fork, point B in figure 7.7. I give you another bit of information (right), again conveyed as a binary digit (0), that allows you to choose the correct road again. Each bit you receive allows you to choose between two roads. Because there are four roads you could have chosen from when you started at A (two leading from B and two from the fork below B), two bits of information allow you to choose from among four (equally likely) possible alternatives.

You keep on strolling down that road and come to yet another fork (so it is in life), marked C in figure 7.7. Yet another bit of information (right = 0) allows you to choose the correct road again, leading to the point marked D. There are eight destinations you could have chosen from when you started at A, so three bits allow you to choose from among eight (equally likely) possible alternatives. Let's summarize your brief journey:

• If you have one bit of information then you can choose from two (equally likely) possible alternatives (i.e., 2^1).
• If you have two bits of information then you can choose from four (equally likely) possible alternatives (i.e., 2^2).
• Finally, if you have three bits of information then you can choose from eight (equally likely) possible alternatives (i.e., 2^3).

By now you should have spotted a pattern: if you have n bits of information then you can choose from $m = 2^n$ equally likely alternatives. This is somewhat like the game of "20 questions," which allows you (the astute questioner) to discover which one out of about a million ($2^{20} = 1,048,576$) equally possible objects is in the mind of your opponent. Conversely, it follows that, if you have to choose between m equally likely alternatives then you need $n = \log_2 m$ bits of information in order to choose correctly (using logarithms to the base 2 makes it easier to interpret such equations).

Bits, Binary Digits, and Entropy

There is a subtle, but important, difference between a bit and binary digit. A binary digit is a zero or a one, whereas a bit is an *amount of information*, which can be conveyed by a binary digit or, more generally, by any symbol or word (e.g., yes/no). To give an extreme example, if you already know that you should take the left road from point A in figure 7.7, and if I show you the binary digit 1 (i.e., left) then I have given you a binary digit, but I have provided you with no information. Thus, because you already knew which way to go at the first fork, I only need give you *n-1* bits of information for you to navigate *n* forks.

To explore this idea fully, consider two more examples. Suppose you know that there is a 50 percent chance that the left road is correct. Because both alternatives are equally probable, you know from the previous section that the binary digit I show you (1) provides exactly one bit of information. For the final example, suppose there's a 90 percent chance that the left road is correct, in which case the binary digit that I show you (1) provides more than zero, but less than one, bit of information. Given these probabilities, you wouldn't be surprised to learn that the left road is correct, but you *would* be surprised to learn that the right road is correct. In fact, the amount of information you receive is the same as your degree of *surprise* regarding each alternative. But how can we measure the degree of surprise?

Claude Shannon proved in 1949 that the amount of surprise associated with the value of any symbol s (such as a binary digit) is $H = \log_2 1/p(s)$, where $p(s)$ denotes the probability of a specific value of s, and H is now known as "Shannon information" (Shannon & Weaver 1949). If $s = 1$ (a value that occurs with probability 0.9), and we substitute this into Shannon's equation, then we obtain $H = \log_2 1/0.9 = 0.152$ bits. In other words, if there is a 90 percent probability that the correct road to choose is left (1), and if I tell you that, indeed, the left road is correct on this occasion then you should be relatively unsurprised, and this is reflected in the small amount of information you have gained (0.152 bits). In contrast, the surprise (Shannon information) associated with the value $s = 0$—the *right* road is correct—is $H = \log_2 1/0.1 = 3.322$ bits, where this large number again reflects the amount of surprise associated with this unexpected alternative. If we measure the information provided by these two different alternatives over a long time period then we would find that the *average* information supplied by both alternatives is 0.469 bits. This is because one alternative is 9 times more probable than the other, and because it occurs 9 times as often, the relatively small surprise values associated with that alternative ($s = 1$) will dominate the average. The average Shannon information provided by a variable such as s is known as the "entropy" of s.

More generally, if you have *any* information about which alternative to choose then this can be of benefit in two different ways. First, as we have just seen, you need to be given fewer than n bits of information to navigate n forks in the road. Second, you can negotiate more than n forks by combining your own information with the n bits of information you receive. This will prove important later when we consider the recoding that ganglion cells may provide.

Photoreceptors as Information Channels

Now suppose we divide up the possible output voltages of a photoreceptor into eight disjoint (i.e., non-overlapping) intervals or *bins* between 1 and 80 mV, as in figure 7.8 (this is not the actual range, but let's pretend it is to keep things simple). Initially, you've no idea which bin contains the photoreceptor voltage is in. If you ask me whether the output is more than 40 mV (i.e., in the top four bins, 5–8), then my answer will tell you which half of the voltage range contains the photoreceptor output. If my answer takes the form of a binary digit (0 = "no" and 1 = "yes") and if you've no prior information, then it (1)—yes, it is—provides you with one bit of information. This leads you from voltage fork A to voltage fork B in figure 7.8.

So now you know the voltage must be in the range 41–80 mV and must therefore correspond to one of the four voltage bins marked 5–8. Similarly,

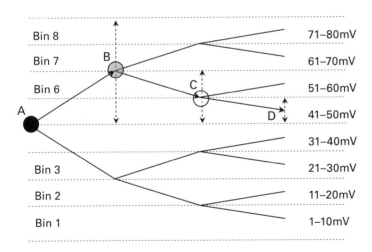

Figure 7.8
If the output voltage of a cone is divided into eight levels or bins then three bits* are sufficient to specify which one of eight possible voltage bins it's in (bin number 5 here). By analogy with figure 7.7, this destination bin could be reached through three decision points, at A, B, and C.

knowing which path to take from fork A in the road of figure 7.7 ultimately committed you to one subset of four out of eight possible destinations. Now, within the range of 41–80 mV (the subset of bins 5–8), if you ask me whether the output is more than 60 mV (the mid-point of the range 41–80 mV), then my answer tells you which half (either 41–60 or 61–80 mV) contains the photoreceptor output. My answer (0)—no, it's not—leads you to the voltage fork C in figure 7.8.

Having arrived at the final voltage fork C, there are just two bins left (bins 5 and 6, with ranges 41–50 and 51–60 mV). If you ask me whether the output is more than 50 mV (the mid-point of the range 41–60 mV) then my answer tells you which half of the voltage range 41–60 mV contains the photoreceptor output. My answer (0)—no, it's not—leads you to point D in figure 7.8, which tells you which of the eight bins (bin 5) the cone output value resides in.

Of course, this could go on indefinitely, and because each binary digit provides one bit*, each additional bit would *halve* your uncertainty about the cone voltage value. (The asterisk [*] after "bit" or "bits" is a reminder that a binary digit [0 or 1] corresponds to one bit of information only if the two alternatives [roads, voltage bins] under consideration are *equally* probable.) Equivalently, each additional bit doubles the number of possible voltage bins that can be discriminated, and therefore halves the voltage range spanned by each bin. Thus, if you specify a photoreceptor voltage using eight bits then that voltage is one out of 256 (i.e., 2^8) possible values. For comparison, because you can adequately specify the intensity of each pixel in a digital image with eight bits, its intensity has one out of 256 possible values between 0 and 255, as shown in figure 2.14.

Even after receiving the three bits* of information in the form of the binary string [1 0 0] (or eight bits or even 1,000 bits), you still don't know the *exact* output voltage of a given photoreceptor. But you get to know more about it as the number of bins increases because this effectively decreases the voltage range spanned by each bin.

The point of all this is that a photoreceptor or a neuron is essentially an information channel. This means that it has a finite capacity, so we can squeeze only so much information through it. For a photoreceptor, this information takes the form of its output voltage, as we have seen in the example above. For a neuron (e.g., a ganglion cell), information usually takes the form of action potentials or spikes, for reasons discussed in chapter 3 (see "Action Potentials, Telephone Cables, and Information Spikes"). For simplicity, we will assume that it is the firing rate or number of spikes per second that carries the information, although the precise timing of action potentials can also carry information (Rieke et al. 1997). Just as different voltage bins can be used to specify the output voltage of a photoreceptor, so different firing rate bins can be used to specify the output of a neuron. Because each spike forces the release of small packets of chemical messengers (neurotransmitters) at a synapse, the amount of messenger received by the post-synaptic neuron acts as an indicator of the firing rate. In one case (photoreceptors), each bin specifies a range of voltages; in the other (ganglion cells), each bin specifies a range of firing rates. But, in both cases, the larger the number of bins, the more precisely the state of a photoreceptor or neuron can be measured. And when considered as information channels, the larger the number of bins, the more information can be squeezed along each channel.

Bits and Bins in the Visual System

Having established that the amount of information is related to the "number of bins," we should say a little about what these bins might correspond to in the visual system. Basically, the effective number of bins is determined by the number of *discriminable states* of a photoreceptor or neuron. Consider the imaginary photoreceptor above with an output between 1 and 80 mV that feeds into a ganglion cell (neuron). Now assume the ganglion cell's firing rate is at baseline when the photoreceptor has an output of 1 millivolt and fires at its maximum rate when the photoreceptor's output is anywhere in the range 2–80 mV. So, by observing the ganglion cell's firing rate, we can tell only whether the photoreceptor's output is at 1 mV ("off") or between 2 and 80 mV ("on"). It is as if the ganglion cell effectively categorizes the photoreceptor output into one of two voltage bins because it can only discriminate between two photoreceptor states.

A more sensitive or discriminating ganglion cell might have a steady firing rate of 10 spikes per second for all photoreceptor outputs between 1 and 10 mV, 20 spikes per second for all photoreceptor outputs between 11 and 20 mV, and so on, until a maximum firing rate of 80 spikes per second is reached, for all photoreceptor outputs between 71 and 80 mV. This ganglion cell effectively recodes the photoreceptor output voltage into eight distinct states, each of which corresponds to one voltage bin. If these eight states occur with equal probability then the ganglion cell's firing rate provides exactly three bits of information about the photoreceptor state.

In practice, the firing rates of ganglion cells don't jump between, say, 10 spikes per second and 20 spikes per second but instead vary continuously between zero and 100 spikes per second. But, without going into the details, the logic that underpins the example given here can also be applied to continuous voltages and firing rates.

Of course, this line of reasoning also applies to the photoreceptor itself, which effectively recodes luminance levels in the retinal image to voltage levels in the photoreceptor's output. It follows that the sensitivity of a photoreceptor determines how many discriminable states it can be in, which determines the amount of information it can convey about light levels in the retinal image.

What a Waste

As already noted, adjacent red and green cones usually have voltages that are similar, so that almost all the information conveyed by the red cone's output is also given by the green cone's output. This might mean, for example, that whenever the red cone's output lies in the fifth voltage bin, the green cone's output usually lies in the fourth or sixth bin (for simplicity, we'll ignore the possibility that the green cone's output could also lie in the fifth bin).

More generally, whenever the red cone's output lies in one voltage bin, the green cone's output usually lies in an adjacent bin. Thus, if we know the voltage bin of the red cone then we know that the green cone's output lies in a bin either above or below this. So if I tell you that the red cone's output lies in the fifth bin then you know that the green cone's output lies in either the fourth or sixth voltage bin. In other words, given that the three bits of information conveyed by the red channel tell you which of eight bins the red cone output is in, you need exactly one extra bit* of information to determine which of two possible states the green cone is in. If I provide that extra bit, by telling you to add (1) or subtract (0) one bin from the one you already know about then you would have received a total of four bits of information (three bits for the red cone, plus one extra bit for the red – green [red minus green] cone difference).

So, in this case, a total of just four bits is sufficient to specify which of eight voltage bins is occupied by each of two photoreceptors. But we know that each channel has three bits' worth of capacity, making a total of 3 + 3 = 6 bits worth of capacity. The similarity in the red and green cone outputs means there are a total of just four bits of information, even though six *binary digits* are used to carry these four *bits*. The "missing" two bits of information have been wasted by sending two very similar messages down the red and green information channels. This waste can be reduced, and even eliminated, if we can find a way to recode the messages so that they are no longer similar to each other.

The similarity between messages or signals is measured in terms of a quantity called the "correlation." For example, if the value of the red cone's output can be predicted from the value of the green cone's output then they have a high correlation; conversely, if the value of the red cone's output cannot be predicted at all from the value of the green cone's output then they have zero correlation and are said to be "uncorrelated." Clearly, if the brain used one ganglion cell to send each cone's output to the LGN then ganglion cells connected to red and green cones would have highly correlated outputs. But if we could share out the red and green cone's outputs between two ganglion cells then it might be possible to produce ganglion cells with outputs that are uncorrelated. This would make full use of the information capacity of each ganglion cell because they would not be conveying almost the same information.

Sum-Difference Recoding
One simple way to ensure that the outputs of two ganglion cells are uncor-related consists of using one cell to carry the *sum* of the red and green cone outputs, and another to carry the *difference* between their outputs, as in figure 7.9 (plate 18). For brevity, let's call this type of recoding a

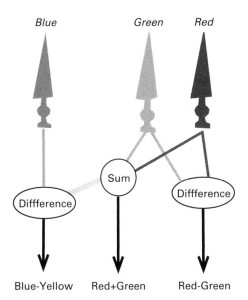

Figure 7.9 (plate 18)
Combining cone outputs to produce three color information channels. The red + green channel is known as the "luminance channel." From Frisby & Stone 2010.

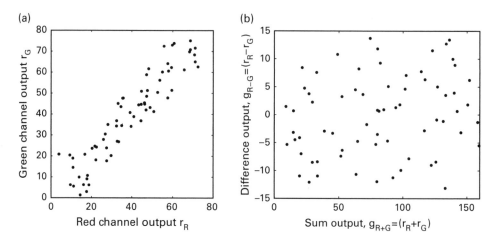

Figure 7.10

Schematic illustration of recoding channel outputs efficiently using sum-difference recoding. (a) The similar tuning curves of red and green channels (e.g., cones) ensures that nearby cones have similar (correlated) output values, r_R and r_G, as indicated by the cloud of points close to the diagonal. (b) These can be recoded as the sum $g_{R+G} = r_R + r_G$ and difference $g_{R-G} = r_R - r_G$ channels (e.g., ganglion cells), which have outputs that are not correlated, as indicated by the uniform coverage of dots in a graph of g_{R+G} versus g_{R-G}.

"sum-difference recoding." A way to check whether these sum and difference signals are correlated is to see if one can be *predicted* from a knowledge of the other. For example, if the two cone outputs are represented as r_R and r_G then knowing the value r_R tells us roughly what value r_G has, as shown in figure 7.10a. For example, figure 7.10a indicates that, if $r_R = 40$ mV, then the value of r_G also has a value of about 40 mV, because most of the data points cluster around the diagonal.

Now, supposing that these values were recoded in terms of a sum ganglion cell output $g_{R+G} = r_R + r_G$ and a difference ganglion cell output $g_{R-G} = r_R - r_G$, as shown in figure 7.10b (note that r denotes cone photoreceptor output, whereas g denotes ganglion cell output). In this case, figure 7.10b indicates that, if $g_{R+G} = 100$ mV (for example) then the corresponding heights of points value of g_{R-G} could have any value, because the data points are uniformly distributed all over the graph.

Using this sum-difference recoding, if you know the value of the sum ganglion cell output g_{R+G} then what can you infer about the value of the difference ganglion cell output g_{R-G}? This is like saying, "If you know that two numbers sum to 100, what can you infer about the difference between them?" When the question is put like this, the answer is clearly "Nothing at all" because both numbers could be 50, or one could be 50.1 and the other 49.9, or 50.2 and 49.8, or any of an infinite series of number pairs that summed to 100. Thus, using this recoding, knowing the value of the sum ganglion cell output g_{R+G} (e.g., 7) tells you nothing about the value of the difference ganglion cell output g_{R-G} and vice versa. In other words, knowing the value of *one* ganglion cell output tells you *nothing* about the value of the *other* ganglion cell output—an unequivocal indication that the outputs of the sum and difference ganglion cells are uncorrelated. But this implies that recoding cone outputs in terms of sums and differences ensures the brain could, in principle, make full use of the capacity of ganglion cells as information channels. The approximate outputs of these hypothetical sum and difference channels are shown in figure 7.11 (plate 19).

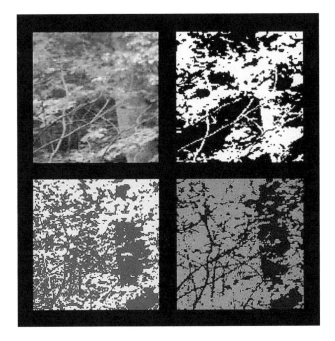

Figure 7.11 (plate 19)
Idealized version of the output of three color channels defined in figure 7.9 (plate 18), based on an original image (top left). The output of the red + green or luminance (upper right), blue − yellow (lower left), and red − green (lower right) channels. Reproduced with permission from Cronin, Ruderman, & Chiao 1998.

Recoding and Efficient Coding

In theory, sum-difference recoding could be used either to reduce the overall number of ganglion cells required or to specify the output voltages (states) of photoreceptor cells with greater precision. In other words, more information translates to a larger number of photoreceptor voltage bins, which means that each bin spans a smaller range of photoreceptor voltages. In reality, the retina may have achieved both of these possibilities because the information from the 126 million photoreceptors in the retina is translated (albeit imperfectly) into the outputs of one million ganglion cells of the optic nerve, and these ganglion cells seem to use sum-difference recoding.

In our example, before sum-difference recoding, each ganglion cell transmitted three bits about one photoreceptor. But, because both red and green cone photoreceptors had similar states, some of the information transmitted by the two ganglion cells was the same. This wasted some capacity, which we assumed to be two bits, so the total amount of information transmitted by the two ganglion cells was only four bits. In other words, even though the total capacity of the two ganglion cells is six bits, the amount of information transmitted by them *about the photoreceptor states* was only four bits. This quantity is known as the "mutual information" between the states of the ganglion cells and the states of the photoreceptors that act as inputs to the ganglion cells. This, in turn, implies that (after recoding) the total available channel capacity of six bits could be used to specify the state of each photoreceptor with greater precision (i.e., using more than eight bins per photoreceptor).

We already know that a total of four bits can specify each of two correlated photoreceptor states down to a precision of one out of eight possible voltage bins. We also know that the recoding example above frees up two (= 6 − 4) extra bits, or one bit per channel. How could the extra bit per channel help? Well, as we have seen above, each additional bit *doubles* the number of voltage bins, so having one extra bit per channel allows the number of voltage bins per channel to be increased from eight to sixteen. In effect, the correlation between channels allows us to use sum-difference recoding of photoreceptor states, so that each photoreceptor state can be specified as one out of sixteen possible voltage bins.

In summary, even though red and green cone photoreceptors each transmit three bits, the correlation between the photoreceptor states means, together, they transmit a total of only four, rather than six, bits of information about their voltage states. However, after sum-difference recoding (e.g., within ganglion cells), the amount of information conveyed about the correlated photoreceptor states increases from four to six bits. Given the degree of correlation under consideration here, this means that (before recoding) each photoreceptor state can be specified to one out of eight possible voltage bins, whereas (after recoding) each photoreceptor state can be specified to one out of sixteen possible voltage bins.

Ganglion Cells as Information Channels

How does the above theoretical analysis tally with the ganglion cells observed in the retina? First, each parasol retinal ganglion cell (see p. 101), which projects to the magnocellular layer of LGN, has an output that is the *sum* of *red and green cone* outputs. Second, each midget retinal ganglion cell, which projects to the parvocellular layer of LGN (see "Magno, Parvo, and Konio Layers in the LGN" in chapter 4), has an output that is the *difference* between *red and green cone* outputs in the fovea, as shown in figure 7.12 (plate 20). (Different cells carry only red – green or only green – red signals.) Within the periphery, however, each midget retinal ganglion cell has an output that is the *sum* of red and green cone outputs.

Thus *both* the parasol and midget retinal ganglion cells seem to contribute to the red + green channel, whereas only midget retinal ganglion cells contribute to the red – green channel. Because a combination of red and green light appears yellow, the red + green channel can be considered as

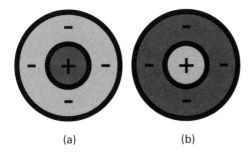

(a)   (b)

Figure 7.12 (plate 20)
Schematic diagram of typical receptive fields of red/green center-surround ganglion cells. (a) Red light in the center excites this cell, whereas green in the annulus inhibits it. As the ganglion cell is connected mainly to red-sensitive cones in the center, and mainly to green-sensitive cones in the annulus, this cell shows a spatial red/green opponency, analogous to the luminance opponency shown in figure 3.23. (b) Green light in the center excites this cell, whereas red in the annulus inhibits it.

a yellow channel, and because it measures overall light levels it is traditionally known as the "luminance channel." In contrast, the difference between red and green cone outputs corresponds to a channel in which red and green act in opposition to each other (e.g., red increases the channel's output, whereas green decreases it) and is called the "red – green opponent channel." Note that the particular sign of this opponency is not important, because, for example, red – green (i.e., red minus green) is the same as –(green – red), so if we know one of these then the other is easily obtained. However, the neuronal mechanism that encodes the difference may involve both red – green and green – red ganglion cells, as described below.

The output of each *bistratified* retinal ganglion cell, which projects to the konio layers of LGN, corresponds roughly to the *difference* between *blue channel (cone)* outputs and the yellow channel (i.e., the *sum* of the *red and green cone* outputs), $g_{B-RG} = r_B - (r_R + r_G)$, as shown in figure 7.13 (plate 21). (Different cells carry only blue – yellow (red + green) or only yellow – blue signals.) Because there's some overlap between the tuning curves of the cones that make up the blue and yellow channels, their outputs are correlated. Without going into the details, recoding these as a difference signal g_{B-RG} ensures that each of the three channels defined above is uncorrelated with the other two. Thus the three cone outputs (red, green, and blue) can be converted into three combinations (blue-yellow, yellow, and red-green), each of which seems to be carried by a different type of ganglion cell.

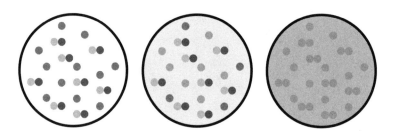

Figure 7.13 (plate 21)
Schematic diagram of typical receptive field of a bistratified retinal ganglion cell, which is excited by blue light and inhibited by yellow light. (Left) Yellow channel is represented by pairs of red and green cones, and the number of blue-sensitive cones is about the same as the combined number of red- and green-sensitive cones in this example. (Middle) Yellow light excites the red/green receptors, which have inhibitory connections to the ganglion cell. (Right) Blue light excites the blue receptors, which have excitatory connections to the ganglion cell.

Once we (or our brains) have received the recoded signals as output values of ganglion cells, we could recover the red, green, and blue channel (cone) outputs by adding or subtracting ganglion channel outputs from each other. For example, the green channel output could be obtained by subtracting the difference channel $g_{(R-G)} = r_R - r_G$ from the yellow (luminance) channel $g_{RG} = r_R + r_G$, and dividing by 2, which yields $r_G = [(r_R = r_G) - (r_R - r_G)]/2$. Similarly, the red channel output could be obtained by adding the difference channel g_{R-G} to the yellow channel g_{R+G}, as $r_R = [(r_R - r_G) + (r_R + r_G)]/2$.

The essential thing is that the information regarding cone outputs is implicit in the ganglion cell outputs, and that it can be encoded to use the full capacity of the ganglion cells as information channels. Thus sending the output values of, say, red and green cones in separate ganglion cells would waste the channel capacity of ganglion cells, whereas sum-difference recoding would not. One result of this is that each cone's outputs could be recovered more accurately (i.e., with greater precision) within the LGN or striate cortex.

Principal Component Analysis

You might well ask why we decided to recode the cone outputs in terms of sums and differences. One answer would be "Because that's what ganglion cells seem to do." However, a more principled answer is "Because that is one recoding that preserves as much information as possible about cone outputs. Indeed, there is a method called "principal component analysis" (PCA), which, under mild assumptions, finds a recoding of cone outputs that preserves as much information as possible. When PCA is applied to model cone outputs obtained in response to naturalistic images, the resultant recoding yields three channels that are qualitatively similar to the three color channels described above (figures 7.9 and 7.11, plates 18 and 19; Cronin, Ruderman, & Chiao 1998), although the results can depend on the precise nature of the cone model used (Simoncelli & Olshausen 2001).

Noise

All of this would work perfectly well were it not for the ubiquitous curse of information transmission in computers, telephone wires, and brains—noise. Whatever its cause (and there are many), noise materializes as a form jitter in the level of a signal, whether the voice amplitude in a telephone wire, the voltage that tells your computer you just typed a letter, the output voltage of a cone photoreceptor, the amount of neurotransmitter arriving at a synapse, or the firing rate of a neuron. In every case, the effect of noise is to limit the amount of information that can be transmitted through a given information channel.

In the case of the eye, noise is added by stray photons of light hitting photoreceptors, by thermally induced spontaneous changes in the light-sensitive chemical in each photoreceptor, by the randomness with which released neurotransmitter diffuses across a synapse, and by the variable delay induced by the imperfect transmission of a spike along each axon. All of these processes add uncertainty to the message received by the brain, specifically, by neurons in the LGN receiving the outputs of retinal ganglion cells.

At low levels of noise, the sum-difference recoding described in the previous section boosts the available capacity above that obtainable without recoding. In contrast, at high levels of noise, sum-difference recoding can actually *reduce* the available channel capacity, in which case a form of pure summation should be used in principle with respect to center-surround ganglion cells (see "Push-Pull Amplifiers in the Brain?" in chapter 3; see also "Further Reading"). On the other hand, the detailed experiments required to establish a similar effect with respect to color processing have not yet been done.

More Pushing and Pulling?

We have implicitly assumed that the difference between two cone types can be indicated by the output of a single ganglion cell. However, on page 69, we discovered that the difference between two outputs can be either positive or negative, but that firing rates cannot. We also learned that this problem can be solved by using push-pull pairs of on-center and off-center ganglion cells in tandem.

We can apply the same logic here to obtain push-pull pairs of red – green ganglion cells. Specifically, one ganglion cell in each pair would have an output that increases when the red – green difference (i.e., $r_R - r_G$) between red and green cones goes above zero, and the other member of each pair would have an output that increases when this difference goes below zero (analogous to figure 3.24). In principle, these cells could project to a hypothetical composite red – green cell with an output that is always positive and that increases in proportion to the difference $r_G - r_R$. Even though there is no direct evidence for the pairing of individual cells, ganglion cells for both red – green and for blue – red/green differencing operations exist. As before, such composite cells would not only take care of how to encode positive and negative differences in cone outputs; each of them would also provide a combined output that is more linear than would otherwise be obtained.

Color Aftereffects

In the opening paragraph to this chapter, we asked why looking at red yields a green aftereffect, whereas looking at yellow yields a blue aftereffect, as in figure 7.1 (plate 12). Now we can see that the recoding that begins in the retina creates a red – green channel and a blue – yellow channel. If, as seems likely, each channel is implemented as pairs of push-pull cells, then this may account or the aftereffects observed. These effects are conventionally described in terms of "red/green" and "blue/yellow opponent processes."

Prolonged exposure to red may differentially reduce activity in the ganglion cells that take care of the positive part of the red – green channel (perhaps by fatigue), while having little impact on the ganglion cells that take care of the negative part of the red – green channel. Thus, after a red disk is removed from view, there's an imbalance in the relative activity of the red – green versus the green – red ganglion cells. The brain can interpret the reduced activity in the red – green ganglion cells as signaling the presence of green, which may explain why looking at red yields a green aftereffect. The same type of argument can be applied to account for the blue – yellow aftereffect in figure 7.1.

The coding of color into three channels seems to extend beyond the ganglion cells, into LGN and even beyond striate cortex, so we can't be certain about the location of the cells that mediate these aftereffects. But we can be fairly sure that the nature of the process responsible for them involves the red – green and blue – yellow channels.

Now that we have some idea of how to recode cone outputs so that the brain can receive accurate information regarding their states, we will back up somewhat and explore why the cones may have such apparently peculiar tuning curves.

Are Cone Tuning Curves Optimal?

Accounting for the massive overlap between the tuning curves of the red and green cones has always presented a challenge to vision scientists. In bright sunshine, the red and green cone outputs contain relatively little noise, so the red + green channel gives an accurate measure of the luminance in each part of the retinal image. Because the red and green cones have such similar tuning curves, adding red and green cone outputs gives an accurate measure of the amount of light, or luminance, at each point in the retinal image. And because these summed outputs are often part of a center-surround receptive field, they can also contribute to an accurate measure of local contrast, and they can do so even for relatively fine details (i.e., at high spatial frequencies), as in figure 3.21. However, under low-light conditions, the outputs of the red and green cones become increasingly noisy. Under these conditions, adding the red and green cone outputs reduces the impact of noise. Thus the overlapping tuning curves of the red and green cones contribute to vision at fine spatial scales in good lighting conditions, and reduce the impact of noise under low-light conditions.

In contrast, the opponent red – green channel carries chromatic information regarding the relative proportions of red and green wavelengths of light. But the difference between the red and green cone outputs is necessarily smaller than their sum, making this red – green channel more susceptible to the effects of noise than the red + green channel, especially in low-light conditions. Under good lighting conditions, when the effects of noise are minimal, this opponent red – green channel effectively carries chromatic information regarding red/green wavelengths.

Thus the overlapping tuning curves represent a compromise between the brain's need for accurate spatial information at fine spatial scales and its need for accurate chromatic information. A large overlap between the tuning curves of the red and green cones gives accurate spatial information at the cost of more noisy chromatic information. Conversely, a smaller overlap gives good chromatic information at the cost of more noisy spatial information (Lewis & Zhaoping 2006). This may explain the absence of blue cones in the fovea, where spatial acuity may take precedence over chromatic accuracy.

Simplifications

The above account includes many simplifications, which were made for the most part to construct a transparent and accessible account, without affecting the nature of the core ideas being expressed. Some of the most notable simplifications are as follows.

First, we have largely ignored the fact that there are almost no blue cones in the fovea, which reduces image distortion due to *chromatic aberration* (see figure 2.8).

Second, we have assumed that each cone can signal only eight distinct output levels at a rate of three bits* per second, a number that is certainly too low. In fact, each ganglion cell transmits information about the inputs it receives from photoreceptors at a rate between 0.5 to 41.2 bits per second

(Nirenberg et al. 2001; for estimates of the information associated with neurons in different sensory systems, see Rieke et al. 1997, p. 100).

Third, we have ignored the fact that the midget and parasol ganglion cells usually have center-surround receptive fields, and that the bistratified cells that signal blue – yellow differences do not. This lack of a center-surround structure is probably due to the relatively large amounts of noise in blue cone outputs, the effects of which are reduced by taking a spatial average.

Fourth, we have glossed over the distinction between two parameters being "uncorrelated" and being "independent" parameters. For our purposes, this is not a crucial distinction, but it will matter for readers who wish to delve more deeply into the papers listed in "Further Reading." Basically, being uncorrelated can be viewed as a weak form of independence.

And fifth, we have ignored the fact that the output of a photoreceptor approximates a logarithmic function of the amount of light captured by that photoreceptor. This logarithmic encoding seems to be a universal property of photoreceptors, which allows their outputs to span the enormous range of luminance levels encountered in different lighting conditions.

This foray into the realms of efficient coding and information-theoretic accounts of visual processing is necessarily incomplete in an introductory text. The account given here represents the foothills of the overall framework, and hopefully provides a glimpse of the mountain ranges beyond, which are left for the reader to explore. Above all, the particular information-theoretic account given here represents one example of the benefits of a computational analysis of the problems faced by the brain in its efforts to work out what in the world caused the retinal image.

8   A Hole in the Head

"But I don't want to go out among mad men," said Alice. "Ah, but you can't help it," said the cat. "We're all mad here."
—Lewis Carroll, *Alice's Adventures in Wonderland*

Impressions

What is that? Neither colored nor moving, yet not gray nor still. Neither big nor animal, yet not small nor human. Perhaps, after all, it is merely the thing itself.

Forms of Blindness

We see the world in terms of particular visual properties or physical parameters such as color, motion, depth, orientation, and texture. Indeed, we saw in chapter 4 how different brain regions or cell types seem to specialize in the processing of different parameters. What would the world seem like if our ability to see one of these parameters was suddenly removed?

In 1986, the neurologist Oliver Sacks received the following letter:

I am a rather successful artist just past 65 years of age. On January 2nd of this year I was driving my car and was hit by a small truck on the passenger side of my vehicle. When visiting the emergency room of a local hospital, I was told I had a concussion. While taking an eye examination, it was discovered that I was unable to distinguish letters or colors. The letters appeared to be Greek letters. My vision was such that everything appeared to me as viewing a black and white television screen. Within days, I could distinguish letters and my vision became that of an eagle—I can see a worm wriggling a block away. The sharpness of focus is incredible. BUT—I AM ABSOLUTELY COLOR BLIND. I have visited ophthalmologists who know nothing about this colorblind business. I have visited neurologists, to no avail. Under hypnosis I still can't distinguish colors. I have been involved in all kinds of tests. You name it. Color TV is a hodge-podge. . . . (Sacks & Wasserman 1996, p. 3)

Various clinical tests confirmed that the artist had indeed become completely color blind, that he suffered from an extreme form of what's known as "achromatopsia." For a painter, this was tantamount to Beethoven's descent into absolute deafness in his later years. Unsurprisingly, the artist put aside his color paints and, from then on, produced canvases painted entirely in the "uncolors" of his new gray world. You can get at least some idea of what it might be like to suddenly not be able to see color by turning down the color dial on any digital display until all that's left are shades of gray. However, a deficit that is harder to imagine is losing the ability to see motion.

Josef Zihl, Detlev von Cramon, and Norbert Mai studied a 43-year-old woman who had bilateral damage (i.e., on both sides of the brain) to a region that seems to correspond to area MT (V5), just in front of the occipital lobes. The result of this damage was an inability to perceive motion, called "akinetopsia." Zihl and colleagues reported that their patient "could not cross the street because of her inability to judge the speed of a car, but she could identify the car itself without difficulty. 'When I see the car at first, it seems far away. But then, when I want to cross the road, suddenly the car seems very near'" (Zihl, von Cramon, & Mai 1983).

Although we're used to seeing static images, we're also used to seeing a world filled with motion. The akinetopsia patient, however, reported that objects appeared not to move at all normally but to "jump from one position to the next, with nothing in between." Thus a reasonable simulation of motion blindness might be given by strobe lighting with a relatively long interval of about 1–2 seconds between strobe flashes. This would give the appearance of a static world, which would suddenly change every few seconds, without any intervening motion.

Of course, the most basic of all parameters is space itself. Damage to different parts of the optic pathway results in "holes" or *scotomas* appearing in different parts of the visual field. Indeed, "natural experiments," such as strokes, have played an important role in elucidating the structure of the visual pathway. For example, a stroke that destroys the left optic tract (i.e., after the optic chiasm) effectively removes vision from the left half of both eyes and therefore induces blindness for the right half of the visual world (i.e., the right visual hemifield). Similarly, damage to the left striate cortex (the target of the left optic tract) induces a scotoma in the right visual hemifield. Surprisingly, these scotomas leave victims unaware of their existence. During migraine attacks I would bash my shoulder on

1   2   3   4   5

Figure 8.1
Blind spot is a scotoma we all have. Cover your right eye and focus the left eye on the star. Now fixate each number in turn, while keeping your attention on the star. The star will disappear when you look at one of the numbers, as its image hits the blind spot on your retina.

doorways because I hadn't realized that part of my visual field was now missing.

The fact that a scotoma isn't immediately obvious to the victim seems surprising until we consider the scotoma all of us have: the blind spot (figure 8.1). As mentioned in chapter 2, the outputs of the retinal ganglion cells cross the surface of the retina and gather at one place to form the optic nerve. Because this place can't also contain any photoreceptors, it effectively forms a small region of the retina that's blind. It's quite near to the fovea on the nasal side, and so it ought to be fairly obvious that we're all walking around with a small hole in our vision (well, two holes actually, one for each retina).

The reason that this natural scotoma is not obvious to us is itself not obvious. The conventional explanation is that the brain "fills in" the missing region of an image using information from the area around the blind spot. But this simply tells us what the brain does without explaining *how* the brain does it. From an evolutionary perspective, it would seem to be an advantage to know where the blind spot is at all times. After all, who would want the retinal image of a leopard about to pounce from a tree to be filled in with the foliage that surrounds the leopard? Fortunately, the blind spots of our two eyes don't coincide in the world, so a region in the world that one eye is blind to can be seen by the other. Indeed, the eyes would have to diverge to an unnatural extent to make the two blind spots coincide in the world. If, instead, the blind spot were on the *temporal* side of the fovea then the convergence of the eyes when fixating on a nearby object would occasionally yield a spot on the object to which *both* your eyes were blind. This may partly explain why the blind spot is where it is.

In one of the most tragic "natural experiments," the 1914–18 Great War, the British neurologist George Riddoch noticed that damage to the striate cortex does not result in total blindness. Although striate damage does result in scotomas, which are effectively large blind spots, Riddoch (1917) found that motion even within the scotoma could be detected, which led him to conclude: "Movement may be recognised as a special visual perception." He coined the term *statokinetic dissociation* to describe this curious finding (also known as the "Riddoch phenomenon"), which has effectively been rediscovered in recent decades. Today, the ability to detect motion within scotomas is known as "blindsight," but the exact details of its anatomical origins remain a matter of debate.

If color and motion can be selectively removed from the brain's visual palette, why not other visual parameters, such as line orientation and depth? So far, no deficit in line orientation has been reported. However, Colin Blakemore and Grahame Cooper (1970) found that raising kittens in an environment dominated by vertical lines seems to selectively remove their ability to perceive any lines that aren't vertical or nearly so. Examination of the striate cortex from the cat revealed simple cells with preferred orientations close to vertical only, suggesting a degree of interaction between "nature and nurture."

Riddoch (1917) was alone in reporting the case of a man with damage to the occipital lobe who seems to have had depth blindness: "The most corpulent individual might be a moving cardboard figure, for his body is represented by an outline only. He has colour and light and shade, but still to the patient he has no protruding features: everything is perfectly flat." Although depth blindness is not a well-documented deficit in modern neuropsychology, a particular form of depth blindness, stereoblindness, is. As mentioned previously, about 10 percent of adults can't extract relative depth information from the differences between the images of their eyes. Many of these adults suffered from a squint when they were children, which seems to have prevented development of stereopsis. However, some appear to have recovered at least some degree of stereo vision (see "Stereo Vision" in chapter 5).

So far, we have encountered deficits in the perception of color, motion, depth, stereo, and line orientation (although these last two seemed to be induced by developmental factors). Some deficits, such as color blindness, are associated with damage to a specific area of the cortex but can also be induced by selectively damaging particular cell populations in striate cortex. For example, carbon monoxide poisoning can selectively damage the color-sensitive cells at the centers of singularities in striate cortex. Although Semir Zeki (1993) has suggested that Riddoch's depth-blind patient may have had damage to area V3, the same deficit may result when particular cell types are destroyed. Thus there doesn't have to be a single brain region dedicated to processing a specific visual parameter for that processing to be compromised. Whether a particular function is executed by a specific brain region is an old and fascinating research question, but it's perhaps less important than questions relating to *how* the brain executes any given function.

Gedankenexperiment: Not Carving Nature at Her Joints

Why does the brain choose to slice up the visual world into categories that include color, motion, orientation, and depth? In principle, it could dedicate one subpopulation of neurons to processing upward motions that are red, downward motions that are green, and so on. That might sound silly, but exactly why would it be such a bad idea?

To explore this, let's indulge in a *gedankenexperiment*, a thought experiment, a device that has played a pivotal role in the history of science. Imagine you were the first organism born with a fully formed brain. How should that brain be organized in order to make maximum use of its neurons? Note that the brain does not know anything about the world into which it was born, just as the first brain to evolve knew nothing. It was essentially a *tabula rasa* (blank slate), waiting for evolution to impress upon it the shape of this particular universe. Let's suppose that, in this brave old world, the eye has evolved the ability to detect light and color. What sort of parameters should individual brain cells encode, that is, to what visual properties should they be sensitive?

One option would be to allow each brain cell to decide its own preferred stimulus, provided all possible stimulus values were taken care of in every small region of the retina. Here we'll assume that each small patch of retina has its own dedicated set of subpopulations. You could have, say, four subpopulations to encode different color-motion combinations for each small retinal region: one to encode upward red motion, another to encode downward green motion, a third to encode yellow leftward motion, and a fourth to encode blue rightward motion. But this would mean your brain would be unable to detect red downward, green upward, yellow rightward, or blue leftward motion because it would have no subpopulations of neurons to do so. This can be remedied by adding another four subpopulations: one for red downward motion, another for green upward motion, a third for yellow rightward motion, and a fourth for blue leftward motion. Thus four subpopulations would encode the four possible combinations of red/green vertical (up/down) motion (A in figure 8.2) and another four would encode the four possible combinations of blue/yellow horizontal (left/right) motion (D in figure 8.2).

	Up	Down	Left	Right
Red	A	A	B	B
Green	A	A	B	B
Blue	C	C	D	D
Yellow	C	C	D	D

Figure 8.2
Two-dimensional table of hypothetical subpopulations of neurons, each sensitive to a particular combination of color and motion.

But even these eight subpopulations would *not* encode either *vertical* blue/yellow motion (C in figure 8.2) or *horizontal* red/green motion (B in figure 8.2). To cover these combinations would require another eight subpopulations, making a total of sixteen subpopulations. But even these sixteen would encode motion in only four directions and only four colors. If we wanted to encode five colors and five directions, we would need twenty-five subpopulations, $5 \times 5 = 25$. More generally, if we want to encode N distinct values of each of two parameters then we need a total of $N \times N = N^2$ subpopulations. But this takes care of only two parameters, color and motion. What if the brain also needed to encode information for a third parameter , such as orientation?

To encode three parameters, we would need to add a third axis to the table in figure 8.2 to obtain the reduplicated set of tables shown in figure 8.3. If we needed to encode, say, four distinct values of each parameter, then this would require a total of $4 \times 4 \times 4 = 4^3 = 64$ subpopulations. More generally, if we needed to encode N distinct values of each parameter then we would require a total of $N \times N \times N = N^3$ subpopulations in order to cover all possible combinations of all parameter values.

Even more generally, if we wanted to encode N distinct values of each of k different parameters then we would need to have a total of $M = N^k$ subpopulations of neurons, where each subpopulation encoded a specific combination of the k parameters. This implies that every time the number k of parameters increases by one, the number M of subpopulations increases by a *multiple* of N. For example, if the number of parameters increases from

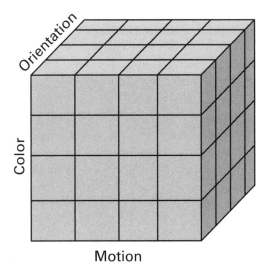

Figure 8.3
Three-dimensional (cube) table of hypothetical subpopulations of neurons, each sensitive to a particular combination of color, motion, and orientation.

three to four, and if each parameter is encoded at ten distinct values, then the number of subpopulations increases from 10^3 (1,000) to 10^4 (10,000). Thus, in what's known as the "curse of dimensionality," the number of subpopulations increases *exponentially* with the number of parameters. Every time we add a new parameter, we have to add a new dimension to the table shown in figure 8.2. And adding one dimension to the two-dimensional table in figure 8.2 yields the three-dimensional cube of figure 8.3, multiplying the number of subpopulations by a factor of 4, (the number of distinct values encoded, in this case) from $4^2 = 16$ to $4^3 = 64$.

Carving Nature at Her Joints

All of this is based on the assumption that subpopulations of neurons choose to encode particular *combinations* of values. What if we were to relax this assumption, and instead allowed each subpopulation to encode just *one* value for each parameter? For example, for color, we could have one subpopulation encode red, another green, a third blue, and a fourth yellow. Similarly, for motion, we could have one subpopulation for each of four distinct directions (up, down, left, right) and, for orientation, one subpopulation for each of four distinct orientations (vertical, horizontal,

45 degrees, and 135 degrees). This would require a total of only 4 + 4 + 4 = 12 subpopulations, which represents a considerable saving compared to the $4 \times 4 \times 4 = 64$ subpopulations given above. With a more realistic number of distinct encoded values for each parameter—ten—the saving is even more dramatic: we would need a "mere" $3 \times 10 = 30$ subpopulations instead of $10^3 = 1,000$.

In essence, this is *why* the brain chooses to encode each physical parameter of the visual world, such as color and motion, in a different subpopulation of neurons: it represents a massive reduction in the number of neurons required. However, this leaves open the question of *how* the evolving brain discovered the separate existence of each of these parameters. After all, there is no reason why the brain should know that there are a number of parameters that effectively lead separate lives in the physical world. This fact must first be discovered, and only then can the brain set about discovering the precise nature of their separate identities.

One way for the evolving brain to discover the separate parameters that describe the visual world is to simply assume they do exist, and then to find a way to determine what they are. The single most important characteristic that defines those visual parameters is that they are *statistically independent* of one another (independence is a generalization of the notion of correlation discussed in chapters 3 and 6). For our purposes, we can consider parameters that are uncorrelated to be independent of one another. For example, because neither the motion nor orientation of an object tells us anything about its color, and vice versa, the parameters of motion, orientation, and color are said to be "statistically independent."

Rather than explicitly seeking out the parameters of color and motion, which the evolving brain couldn't have known about initially, a more general strategy would be to seek out *any* parameters (visual properties) that appear to be statistically independent. Having discovered such a set of parameters, these should make an efficient basis for carving the visual world at its joints. For example, if the different subpopulations encoded the combinations of motion and color given in the example above then cells in the red upward subpopulation would have outputs that were high whenever those in the green downward subpopulation were low, and vice versa. Thus the outputs of each of the two subpopulations can be predicted from the other one, so they cannot, by definition, be independent. (In this example, the two subpopulation outputs have a *negative* correlation, but this is irrelevant; the fact remains that their outputs are not independent.)

If, on the other hand, one subpopulation of cells encoded motion and another encoded color then the outputs of these two subpopulations would be independent because motion and color are themselves independent parameters in the physical world. This also has the desirable side effect of transmitting color and motion data along separate information channels, and as we already know, in order to transmit as much information as possible, idealized (i.e., noise-free) information channels should be statistically independent. So seeking out statistical independence seems to represent a robust strategy for discovering the physical parameters that underpin the structure of the visual world. Indeed, Guillermo Cecchi and colleagues (2010) have found evidence supporting the general idea that color and orientation are statistically independent parameters in the world. So, by discovering and then using statistically independent parameters to encode the retinal image, the brain has essentially discovered the visual properties of motion, color, orientation, and depth and, in so doing, has effectively carved nature at her joints.

Strategies for Object and Face Recognition

When we think of vision, we tend to imagine that its primary purpose is to allow us to recognize objects and faces. Even though recognizing objects and faces is important, especially for social animals like us, vision is essential for many other important actions, as we have seen, from apparently simple tasks like staying vertical to landing a plane.

In the previous pages, we saw how the brain could, over evolutionary time, discover the fundamental physical parameters that underpin the visual world because these coincide with descriptors that are statistically independent. Could a similar strategy be used by the brain to discover objects and faces? If so, the parameters involved would not be those of the simple physical parameters considered above. Instead, they would involve high-order parameters, or features, which must consist of particular combinations of the low-order parameters. The reason for saying "must" is because, once we have considered each of the low-level parameters, the only way to specify visual features is in terms of combinations of low-order parameters. These combinations may be nontrivial, involving more than a simple addition of different parameters, but they are, and can only be, combinations of parameters.

In purely abstract terms, what is it that defines an object or a face? In essence, it is the persistence over time of a set of stable physical parameter values (whether these are high- or low-level parameters). Indeed, it is only by observing how a thing appears to change that its "sameness" can be gauged. Rotating a cup does not alter the cup, but it does alter the cup's appearance. If it is known which parameters characterize a cup when it is viewed from any angle then the cup may be recognized from any viewpoint. So one possible strategy for recognizing an object is to discover the parameters that do not change over time, and to use these as reliable cues to that object's identity.

However, if a cup is rotated before you then the only parameters that do not alter over time are related to its three-dimensional structure. Rotation does not alter the cup's shape nor its color, but even the color of a surface can be reliably estimated only if the 3-D orientation of that surface is known (see figure 5.31).

An alternative proposal by David Marr and Shimon Ullman (1981) that relies only on two-dimensional cues suggests that the brain can identify objects by making use of *characteristic views* of those objects. Such views are relatively stable with respect to changes in viewpoint and imply that recognition occurs through the brain's matching 2-D retinal images to 2-D stored representations of those images, as in figure 8.4. In support of this hypothesis, there's a growing body of evidence that object recognition in humans makes use of characteristic views. This evidence suggests that recognition of an object presented at a particular orientation occurs by matching it to a view that is interpolated (combined) across several stored views of that object.

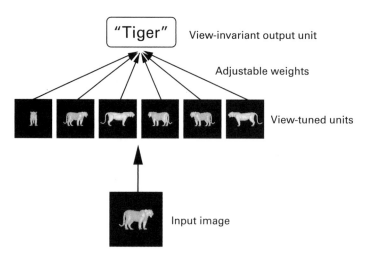

Figure 8.4
Recognition of a tiger from characteristic views.

Both the notion of three-dimensional features that do not alter over time, and two-dimensional characteristic views that change relatively little both require that the brain somehow acquire knowledge of these features or views. To do this, it could simply learn to extract those 3-D features or views that remain stable when all low-level parameter values (e.g., those of motion) are changing. For example, the changing view of a head usually retains certain features such as the eyes and nose, and it's their stability in the retinal image that may allow the brain to adopt as parameters for recognition.

Thus, whereas the brain can discover low-level parameters such as motion and color if it seeks out parameters that are statistically independent of one another, it can discover the high-order parameters of features it needs to recognize objects and faces if it seeks out parameters that change little over time. For low-level parameters, the brain doesn't need to know precisely which parameters underpin the physical world because it will, over evolutionary time, latch onto parameters that are independent of one another. For high-level parameters, the infant brain doesn't need to know what sorts of objects it will encounter because it will latch onto features that remain stable over periods of seconds. This is not intended to deny that some high-order parameters are innate, but simply to note that it would be possible in principle for them to be learned as a side effect of the brain extracting features that remain stable over time.

The finding that similar views of a head are encoded by cells that are near one another is certainly consistent with the general idea just described (see figure 4.20). Similarly, Yasushi Miyashita (1988) found that presenting a monkey with random shapes, but in a fixed order, results in cells near one another responding to shapes that were near one another in the sequence. Thus proximity of shapes in the sequence becomes translated into proximity of cells. Finally, as noted in chapter 4, researchers found that cells that responded to pictures of Jennifer Aniston, of the TV series *Friends*, were close to cells that responded, not to similar faces, but to other characters in the same TV series. In other words, cells that are nearby in cortex responded to features that occurred nearby in time, so that temporal proximity in the world appears to be translated into spatial proximity in the brain.

Evidence of a more circumstantial nature comes from computational modeling studies which suggest that temporal proximity is a powerful strategy for discovering the physical parameters (e.g., 3-D shape, depth, and orientation) that underpin the retinal image (Becker 1996; Foldiak 1991; Stone 1996; Wiskott & Sejnowski 2002). Intriguingly, a side effect of this temporal proximity strategy is that it can also discover parameters that are statistically independent (Stone 2001, 2004), suggesting that the two apparently different strategies outlined above may be intimately related in practice.

Neuropsychology of Object and Face Recognition

Imagine being shown a picture of a pair of spectacles, but all you see is a collection of disconnected parts: a circle, a nose bridge, a bar. No matter how hard you try, the parts refuse to coalesce into a single object. Your reaction might be something like this:

The patient carefully examines the picture of a pair of spectacles shown to him. He is confused and does not know what the picture represents. He starts to guess. "There is a circle . . . and another circle . . . and a stick . . . a cross-bar . . . why, it must be a bicycle?" (Luria 1976)

Patients like Alexander Luria's don't have damage either to their retinas or their striate cortex and can often "see" perfectly well. But they seem to have trouble in integrating information from different parts of the retinal image into a coherent whole. They can usually still identify objects by touch; they just can't recognize them by sight.

For the first three weeks in the hospital the patient could not identify objects when presented visually, and did not know what was on his plate until he tasted it. He identified objects immediately on touching them. When shown a stethoscope he described it as "a long cord with a round thing at the end," and asked if it could be a watch. (Rubens & Benson 1971)

Deficits such as this go under the generic name of "agnosias," of which there are many different types. What these cases demonstrate is that seeing is more than a simple registration of an image on the retina. Indeed, the reaction of someone who has lost the ability to visually recognize objects is somewhat like that of a man who recovered his sight after a lifetime of being blind. Shown a lathe he had always been keen to use, the man could identify only the handle, but when allowed to run his hands over it, he stood back and declared, "Now I've felt it, I can see." (Gregory 1997a, p. 157).

Such cases are astonishing, but our astonishment is born from our own inability to comprehend how someone can't see an object for what it is. In reality, the surprising aspect of such patients is not their inability to recognize objects, but our ability to recognize objects with such apparent ease. As expert perceivers, we have it the wrong way around. It is no more surprising that a person with (or without) brain damage can't recognize an object than that a rock can't recognize an object. What is surprising is that any of us can recognize any object at all.

Recognition deficits are usually associated with damage to nonstriate visual areas. Precisely which areas is a matter of ongoing research, and after a comprehensive review of the literature Martha Farah (2000, p. 103) concluded: "The only generalisation that one can make on the basis of these data is that recognition is a function of the posterior half of the brain!"

In contrast, neurophysiological studies by Charles Gross (1992) and, more recently, imaging studies by others suggest that cells responsive to individual objects and faces can be found in inferotemporal cortex. These cells often show a remarkable degree of selectivity for particular objects (as in figure 8.5, plate 22), and despite changes in the size, contrast, and position of those objects, as shown in figure 8.6.

Cells that respond to different aspects of faces have been found in inferotemporal cortex. These cells seem to be tuned to signal the presence of particular aspects of a face. For example, the cell shown in figure 8.7 responds best to one view of a head, but also responds to a lesser degree to similar views, so that its output gradually diminishes as the head rotates. Other cells have been found that respond to identity, expression, and direction of gaze (Farah 2000).

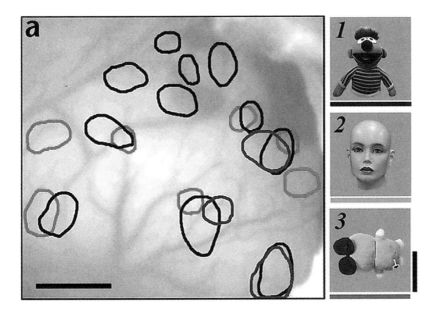

Figure 8.5 (plate 22)
Cells that respond to different objects in area TE, showing spatial distributions of active spots elicited by three different objects. Scale bar in (a): 1 mm.

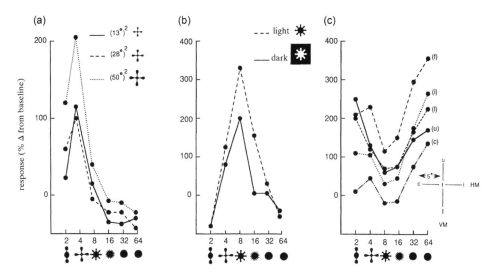

Figure 8.6
Responses of cells in inferotemporal cortex to different objects (noted under x-axis) show similar patterns despite changes in (a) size, (b) contrast, and (c) retinal location. Reproduced with permission from Gross 1992.

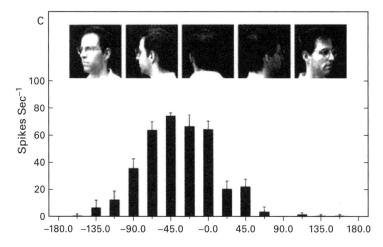

Figure 8.7
Cell in inferotemporal cortex responds selectively to different views of a human head. Reproduced with permission from Logothetis & Sheinberg 1996.

Evidence that images of faces are processed separately from those of other objects comes from individuals who can't recognize faces, even though they can recognize objects in general. Such individuals are said to have "prosopagnosia." A striking case of prosopagnosia involves a man who, after a series of strokes, lost the ability to recognize faces. This so affected his work that he switched careers and became a sheep farmer. Despite his inability to recognize human faces, clinical tests revealed that he recognized each individual one of his sheep's faces (McNeil & Warrington 1993). This suggests that the neural substrate for human face recognition is distinct from that which underpins more general object recognition.

Conclusion

Neuropsychology can tell us which brain regions seem to be involved in specific visual perceptual tasks, for example, that inferotemporal cortex is involved in how the brain sees faces. It can also tell us that different brain regions are involved in processing the images of different types of objects or parameters, for example, MT (V5) seems to be involved in motion perception. But notice that, in almost every instance, we can conclude little more than that a particular brain region is "involved" in some particular task. Of course, this is interesting; indeed, the results from neuropsychological studies are often fascinating. However, the precise nature of the brain's solutions to the many problems of vision cannot be understood only by identifying which brain regions seem to be "involved" in solving those problems. If we want to find out, not only *where*, but precisely *how* a given visual problem is solved by the brain then it seems self-evident that we need to know far more than which region of the brain is involved.

Historically, the relative modularity of function of different brain regions was discovered by "natural experiments" in which a stroke or other trauma effectively knocked out one brain region. These case studies confirm that the brain has clearly chosen to slice up the world along particular lines. More importantly, these lines are not arbitrary. In the case of low-level vision, the brain parcels out visual tasks according to their physical characteristics (e.g., color for V4, motion for V5), but in the case of high-level vision, the brain parcels out visual tasks according to high-order parameters, like objects and faces. Thus, for low-level vision the brain's division of labor respects the physical parameters of the visual world, but for high-level vision this division of labor seems to respect the semantic categories of our everyday experience. In both cases, it seems as if the brain has managed to effectively carve nature at her joints.

9 Brains, Computation, and Cupcakes

Science is built of facts the way a house is built of bricks; but an accumulation of facts is no more science than a pile of bricks is a house.
—Henri Poincaré (1854–1912)

The best science results from asking the right questions, which is much harder than it sounds. However, attempting to answer any old question almost inevitably means starting with the easy ones, and as the answers pile up, the entire exercise seems little more than a form of exotic stamp collecting (having said that, many branches of science began life as a form of "stamp collecting," but matured only with the addition of a coherent theory [e.g., evolution]). With the advent of new experimental techniques, our ability to collect scientific data increases every year. However, our ability to make sense of those data is limited by a single information processing bottleneck, *us*.

Science is essentially a framework for compressing the many and varied observations we make into a neat, and above all, compact theory. Rather than witnessing an ever-increasing amount of data being explained by an ever-decreasing number of competing theories (as occurs in mature sciences like physics), vision science seems to be in a period of data-inflation that is unmatched by a corresponding decrease in the number of theories.

In the year 1900, the mathematician Hilbert proposed a set of key questions which seemed to be at the heart of mathematics. These questions collectively defined the *Hilbert program*, which initiated progress in several fundamental mathematical problems in the years that followed. If ever a scientific discipline were in need of a Hilbert program, it is vision. The main obstacle to such a program is that, unlike mathematics, there is no consensus regarding what the key questions are, nor what approaches are best suited to answering them. But one thing is certain, simply gathering

more data on the details of the visual system, while necessary, is not sufficient for understanding human vision.

A continuation along this path will lead directly into Leibniz's mill (see
chapter 4), and we would then know every detail, but would have little
appreciation of how these details fit together to make a visual system. The
mill was Leibniz's analogy for a brain, because it represented a cutting-edge
technology in his time. Since then, the latest technology has been repeat-
edly used to envisage the workings of the brain, from clockwork dolls
(known as automata), to steam engines (the Watt governor), to telephone
exchanges, to modern computers. In modern terms, we are in danger of
ending up wandering around inside a silicon chip, knowing the inputs and
outputs of every component, but without understanding *how* each component transforms its inputs to outputs, nor *why* such an input-output
transformation is desirable.

David Marr (*Homo computatrix*)

Marr's computational approach makes explicit the distinction between
form and function (which correspond roughly to hardware and computational theory, respectively), as applied to individual neurons, populations
of neurons, and brains. So Marr would be equally happy with a single
computational theory of vision (skipping the algorithmic level for brevity),
whether it was implemented by neurons using spikes as tokens of information, or by frogs passing cupcakes to each other as tokens of information,
provided both of these implemented the same theory. He would, of course,
not be so sanguine about the frogs and cupcakes implementation if anyone
proposed this was how the brain's hardware actually works.

It might be argued that the relative lack of progress made within vision
science using Marr's framework is evidence that it is simply no good.
However, this lack of progress within vision science may be due to a reti-
cence in applying it to the problems of vision. Indeed, even 30 years after
the publication of Marr's book (and more than two decades after this point
was first made by Willshaw and Buckingham [1990]), it seems likely that
Marr is more cited than he is understood. However, so widespread has been
the influence of his ideas that some research fields other than vision (e.g.,
computational neuroscience) take it for granted that a computational
approach is not only desirable, but also necessary, for progress.

As noted previously, to engineers, Marr's framework seems natural,
almost trivial. To neurophysiologists, this framework seems disconnected
from the details of neuronal machinery within the brain. To some psy-

chologists, Marr's framework appears overly formal, too mathematical, and unconcerned with the higher echelons of visual function, like cognition and attention. However, to researchers in the nascent field of computational neuroscience, Marr's ideas represent a radical departure from conventional vision science, a departure which has implications for how we conceive of the brain. The consequences of such a departure are aptly summarized by leading researchers in computational neuroscience: ". . . we claim that the results of a quantitative approach are sufficiently extreme that they begin to alter our qualitative conception of how the nervous system works" (Rieke et al. 1997). This not only follows the general advice given by Galileo in the opening quotation of this book, it also implies that constructing a mathematically precise account of the brain has the potential to change our view of how it works.

Thus, Marr's computational framework has effectively opened the door into a world in which we can consider not merely *how* certain mechanisms (e.g., color and motion opponency) can explain different aspects of visual processing, but more importantly, *why* such mechanisms might be desirable from a computational perspective (e.g., efficient coding which increases information rate and linearity). Once we have gone through this door, we have effectively stepped beyond the confines of nineteenth- and much of twentieth-century visual science. In this brave new world, where computational *reasons* as well as *mechanisms* are accepted as legitimate objects of study, our conception of the nature of scientific explanations should have shifted. For example, the mechanism of mutual inhibition between photoreceptors in the horseshoe crab eye, and the center-surround receptive fields of ganglion cells in the human eye, can both be used to explain *how* luminance edges become exaggerated to yield the Chevreul illusion (see chapter 3). However, only a computational theory provides a plausible explanation of *why* the eyes of both organisms, with their radically different neuronal architectures, should exaggerate luminance edges, and therefore why they should both experience the Chevreul illusion. In essence, we no longer have to accept a mere mechanism as an adequate explanation for a given visual phenomenon; we can now demand that there should also be an underlying *computational reason* for the nature of the information processing provided by that particular mechanism.

Of course, others may disagree with the analysis offered in this chapter, and with the computational perspective adopted throughout much of this book. Only time will tell if this, somewhat personal, viewpoint is justified.

Conclusion

One of the joys of science is that it generates an almost continuous stream of small epiphanies. Occasionally, this stream is interrupted by a larger epiphany, a revolution of the mind, which is not always brought about by a new finding, but by a new way of seeing old facts. Ideas such as Marr's computational framework, information theory, Bayesian analysis, and the efficient coding hypothesis cannot be properly understood without seeing old facts in a new light. Indeed, these intrinsically computational ideas allow us to begin by asking why the visual system is built as it is, and to end by realizing that only a madman would try and build it in any other way. Such a dramatic change in viewpoint is the signature of the best scientific theories. Sadly, such a change in viewpoint is also the mark of absolute delusion. But whereas a delusion fails every test the physical world has to offer, a scientific theory does not.

Further Reading

Readers wishing to expand their understanding of the technical aspects of this book (e.g., in chapters 3, 6, and 7) should read the following eight works (listed below) in roughly this order: Marr 1982, Rieke et al.1997, Stone 2010, Doya et al. 2007, Sivia & Skilling 2006, Cowan 1998, Pierce 1980, and Zhaoping forthcoming.

Bach, M. (2011). Visual phenomena and optical illusions, http://www.michaelbach.de/ot/. Bach's website is dedicated to thought-provoking optical illusions, with a commentary on each one.

Balasubramanian, V., & Sterling, P. (2009). Receptive fields and functional architecture in the retina. *Journal of Physiology, 587*(12), 2753–2767. Information-theoretic analysis of processing in the retina and optic nerve.

Ballard, D. H., & Brown, C. M. (1982). *Computer vision.* Englewood Cliffs, NJ: Prentice-Hall. Available for free online at http://homepages.inf.ed.ac.uk/rbf /BOOKS/ BANDB/bandb.htm. For many years the standard text on computer vision. Although fairly technical, it contains a large amount of tutorial material, especially in the appendices.

Cowan, G. (1998). *Statistical data analysis.* Oxford: Clarendon Press. Complements Devinderit Sivia and John Skillings's book (see below), and they can be read as a pair.

Doya K., Ishii, S., Pouget, A., & Rao, R. P. N. (2007). *Bayesian brain: Probabilistic approaches to neural coding.* Cambridge, MA: MIT Press. This book of edited chapters contains some superb introductions to Bayes' rule in the context of vision and brain function, as well as more advanced material.

Eliasmith, C., & Anderson, C. H. (2004). *Neural engineering: Computation, representation, and dynamics in neurobiological systems.* Cambridge, MA: MIT Press. The idea of using on-center and off-center cells to emulate a push-pull amplifier is described in some detail in this book.

Frisby, J., & Stone, J. V. (2010). *Seeing: The computational approach to biological vision.* Cambridge, MA: MIT Press. Illustrates the use of David Marr's computational framework in the context of visual subdomains (e.g., texture, stereopsis, and motion) and expands on many of the topics covered in *Vision and Brain*.

Gregory, R. L. (1997). *Eye and brain: The psychology of seeing*. 5th ed. Oxford: Oxford University Press. Richard Gregory championed the idea that the brain performs a great deal of inferential work when it interprets an image, and this is reflected in his classic and inspirational book. First published in 1967, the 5th edition was published in 1997.

Hartline, K. (1967). Visual receptors and retinal interaction. In K. Siegbahn et al. (Eds.), *Les Prix Nobel de 1967* (pp. 242–259). Stockholm: Norstedt & Söner. Nobel Lecture. Available for free online at http://nobelprize.org/nobel_prizes/medicine/laureates/1967/hartline-lecture.pdf. A personal account and an accessible review of the mechanisms of vision in the horseshoe crab (*Limulus*).

Hubel, D. (1988). *Eye, brain, and vision*. New York: W. H. Freeman. Available for free online at http://hubel.med.harvard.edu/book/bcontex.htm. Personal account of the visual system, written by one of the founders of modern visual neuroscience. A very readable and insightful book.

Ings, S. (2008). *The eye: A natural history*. London: Bloomsbury. Thorough and engaging popular science introduction to the visual system.

Knight, B. W. (2011). The Hartline-Ratliff model. *Scholarpedia*, 6(1):2121. Available for free online at http://www.scholarpedia.org/article/Hartline-Ratliff_model#Hartline49. Comprehensive summary of the current status of the Hartline-Ratliff model of the horseshoe crab (*Limulus*) eye.

Koch, K., McLean, J., Berry M., Sterling P., Balasubramanian, V., & Freed, M. A. (2004). Efficiency of information transmission by retinal ganglion cells. *Current Biology, 14*, 1523–1530. Neat account of how neurons that fire at different rates convey about the same amount of information per second.

Kolb et al. (2011). *Webvision: The organization of the retina and visual system*. Online book. Available for free at http://webvision.med.utah.edu/book/. Encyclopedic compendium of information on the visual system. In its own words, *Webvision* summarizes recent advances in knowledge and understanding of the visual system through dedicated chapters and evolving discussion to serve as a clearinghouse for all things related to retina and vision science.

Land, M. F., & Nilsson, D. E. (2002). *Animal eyes*. New York: Oxford University Press. Landmark book by two of the most insightful exponents of the intricacies of eye design.

Lettvin, J. Y., Maturana, H. R., McCulloch, W. S., & Pitts, W. H. (1959). What the frog's eye tells the frog's brain. *Proceedings of the Institute of Radio Engineers, 47*,

1940–1951. Groundbreaking paper that brought a computational perspective to bear on the functional architecture of the frog's visual system.

Marr, D. (1982). *Vision: A computational investigation into the human representation and processing of visual information*. Reprint, Cambridge, MA: MIT Press, 2010. Classic inspirational book that articulates the computational framework for vision.

Meister, M., & Berry, M. J. (1999). The neural code of the retina. *Neuron, 22,* 435–450. Accessible review of information processing in the retina.

Nicholls, J. G., Martin, A. R., Wallace, B. G., & Fuchs, P. A. (2001). *From neuron to brain: A cellular and molecular approach to the function of the nervous system*. Sunderland, MA: Sinauer Associates. Classic text on the physiology of neuronal function, well illustrated, clearly written, and with interesting historical comments.

Pierce, J. R. (1961). *An introduction to information theory: Symbols, signals, and noise*. 2nd ed. 1980 New York: Dover. John Pierce writes in an informal, tutorial style but doesn't flinch from presenting the fundamental theorems of information theory.

Reza, F. M. (1961). *An introduction to information theory*. New York: Dover. More comprehensive and mathematically rigorous than John Pierce's book; ideally, it should be read only after first reading Pierce's more informal text.

Rieke, F., Warland, D., van Steveninck, R. R., & Bialek W. (1997). *Spikes: Exploring the neural code*. Cambridge, MA: MIT Press. First modern text to formulate questions about the functions of single neurons in terms of information theory. Superbly written in a tutorial style, well argued, and fearless in its pursuit of solid answers to hard questions. Research papers by these authors, especially those by William Bialek, are highly recommended for their clarity.

Shannon, C. E., & Weaver, W. (1949). *The mathematical theory of communication*. Urbana: University of Illinois Press. Surprisingly accessible book by the founding fathers of information theory. It contains a technical part by Claude Shannon and a discursive part by Warren Weaver.

Sivia, D. S., & Skilling J. (2006). *Data analysis: A Bayesian tutorial*. 2nd ed. Oxford: Clarendon Press. As its title claims, this is indeed a tutorial introduction to Bayesian probability, and an excellent one. The 1996 edition by Devinderit Sivia alone contains the same superb introductory chapters as this edition.

Stone, J. V. (2010). Eyes, flies, and information theory. Tutorial account of a classic three-page paper by Simon Laughlin (1981), which contains a tutorial on information theory. Available for free online at http://jim-stone.staff.shef.ac.uk/papers/laughlin12.pdf.

Zeki Z. (1993). *A vision of the brain.* Oxford: Blackwell. Modern pioneer of visual science Semir Zeki has written a compelling account of the visual functions of different brain regions, with interesting accounts of the historical roots of neuropsychology.

Zhaoping, L. (Forthcoming). *Understanding vision: Theory, models, and data.* Available online at http://www.cs.ucl.ac.uk/staff/Zhaoping.Li/VisionBook.html. Contemporary account of vision based mainly on the efficient coding hypothesis. Even though this book is technically demanding, the introductory chapters give a good overview of the approach.

References

Addams, R. (1834). An account of a peculiar optical phenomenon seen after having looked at a moving body. *London and Edinburgh Philosophical Magazine and Journal of Science, 5*, 373–374.

Adrian, E. D. (1926). The impulses produced by sensory nerve endings: Pt. 1. *Journal of Physiology, 61*, 49–72.

Andrews, S. D., Halpern, T. J., & Purves, D. (1997). Correlated size variations in human visual cortex, lateral geniculate nucleus, and optic tract. *Journal of Neuroscience, 17*(8), 2859–2868.

Atick, J. J., Li, Z., & Redlich, A. N. (1992). Understanding retinal color coding from first principles. *Neural Computation, 4*(4), 559–572.

Atick, J. J., & Redlich, A. N. (1990). Towards a theory of early visual processing. *Neural Computation, 2*(3), 308–320.

Atick, J. J., & Redlich, A. N. (1992). What does the retina know about natural scenes? *Neural Computation, 4*(2), 196–210.

Attneave, F. (1954). Some informational aspects of visual perception. *Psychological Review, 61*(3), 183–193.

Baltrusaitis, J. (1989). *Aberrations: An essay on the legend of forms* (R. Miller, trans.). Cambridge, MA: The MIT Press.

Barlow, H. B. (1953). Summation and inhibition in the frog's retina. *Journal of Physiology, 119*, 69–88.

Barlow, H. B. (1961). Possible principles underlying the transformation of sensory messages. In W. A. Rosenblith (Ed.), *Sensory communication* (pp. 217–234). Cambridge, MA: MIT Press.

Barlow, H. B. (1981). Cortical limiting factors in the design of the eye and the visual cortex. *Proceedings of the Royal Society of London. Series B. Biological Sciences, 212*, 1–34.

Barlow, H. B., Fitzhugh, R., & Kuffler, S. W. (1957). Change of organization in the receptive fields of the cat's retina during dark adaptation. *Journal of Physiology, 137*, 338–354.

Barlow, R. B. (1967). Inhibitory fields in the Limulus lateral eye. Ph.D. diss., Rockefeller University.

Barry, S. (2009). An Interview with "Stereo Sue." *Review of Optometry, 146*(7).

Bayes, T. (1763). An essay towards solving a problem in the doctrine of chances. *Philosophical Transactions of the Royal Society of London, 53*, 370–418.

Becker, S. (1996). Mutual information maximization: Models of cortical self-organisation. *Network:Computation in Neural Systems, 7*(1), 7–31.

Beierholm, U. R., Quartz, S. R., & Shams, L. (2009). Bayesian priors are encoded independently from likelihoods in human multisensory perception. *Journal of Vision, 9*(5), article 23.

Bell, A. H., Hadj-Bouziane, F., Frihauf, J. B., Tootell, R. B., & Ungerleider, L. G. (2009). Object representations in the temporal cortex of monkeys and humans as revealed by functional magnetic resonance imaging. *Journal of Neurophysiology, 101*(2), 688–700.

Bell, A. J., & Sejnowski, T. J. (1995). An information-maximization approach to blind separation and blind deconvolution. *Neural Computation, 7*, 1129–1159.

Berniker, M., Voss, M., & Kording, K. (2010). Learning priors for Bayesian computations in the nervous system. *PLoS ONE, 5*(9), e12686, 09.

Blakemore, C., & Campbell, F. W. (1969). On the existence of neurons in the human visual system selectively sensitive to the orientation and size of retinal images. *Journal of Physiology, 203*, 237–260.

Blakemore, C., & Cooper, G. F. (1970). Development of the brain depends on the visual environment. *Nature, 228*(5270), 477–478.

Blasdel, G. G. (1992). Differential imaging of ocular dominance and orientation selectivity in monkey striate cortex. *Journal of Neuroscience, 12*, 3115–3138.

Bowmaker, J. J., & Dartnall, H. J. A. (1980). Visual pigments of rods and cones in a human retina. *Journal of Physiology, 298*, 501–511.

Brainard, D. H., & Maloney, L. T. (2011). Surface color perception and equivalent illumination models. *Journal of Vision, 11*(5). Available at http://www.journalofvision.org/content/11/5/1.full.pdf+html.

Brainard, D. H., Longere, P., Delahunt, P. B., Freeman, W. T., Kraft, J. M., & Xiao, B. (2006). Bayesian model of human color constancy. *Journal of Vision, 6*(11), 1267–1281.

Brenner, N., Bialek, W., & de Ruyter van Steveninck, R. (2000). Adaptive rescaling maximizes information transmission. *Neuron, 26,* 695–702.

Brewster, D. (1826). On the optical illusion of the conversion of cameos into intaglios, and of intaglios into cameos, with an account of other analogous phenomena. *Edinburgh Journal of Science, 4,* 99–108.

Carandini, M., Heeger, D. J., & Movshon, J. A. (1997). Linearity and normalization in simple cells of the macaque primary visual cortex. *Journal of Neuroscience, 17,* 8621–8644.

Cecchi, G. A., Rao, A. R., Xiao, Y., & Kaplan, E. (2010). Statistics of natural scenes and cortical color processing. *Journal of Vision, 10*(11), article 21.

Clynes, M. (1969). Cybernetic implications of rein control in perceptual and conceptual organization. *Annals of the New York Academy of Sciences, 156,* 629–670.

Coutant, B. E., & Westheimer, G. (1993). Population distribution of stereoscopic ability. *Ophthalmic & Physiological Optics, 13,* 3–7.

Cox, R. T. (1946). Probability, frequency, and reasonable expectation. *American Journal of Physics, 14,* 1–13.

Cronin, T. W., Ruderman, D. L., & Chiao, C. (1998). Statistics of cone responses to natural images: implications for visual coding. *Journal of the Optical Society of America, 15,* 2036–2045.

Darwin, C. (1859). *On the origin of species by means of natural selection, or The preservation of favoured races in the struggle for life.* London: J. Murray.

DeAngelis, G. C., Cumming, B. G., & Newsome, W. T. (2000). A new role for cortical area MT: The perception of stereoscopic depth. In M. S. Gazzaniga (Ed.), *The new cognitive neurosciences* (pp. 305–314). Cambridge, MA: MIT Press.

DeAngelis, G. C., & Newsome, W. T. (1999). Organization of disparity? Selective neurons in macaque area MT. *Journal of Neuroscience, 19*(4), 1398–1415.

de Lange, H. (1958). Research into the dynamic nature of the human fovea-cortex systems with intermittent modulated light: 1. Attenuation characteristics with white and colored light. *Journal of the Optical Society of America, 48,* 777–784.

Deneve, S., Latham, P. E., & Pouget, A. (2001). Efficient computation and cue integration with noisy population codes. *Nature Neuroscience, 4*(8), 826–831.

Derrington, J. V. S. (2001). The lateral geniculate nucleus: A primer. *Current Biology, 11*(16), 635–637.

Dienes, Z. (2008). *Understanding psychology as a science: An introduction to scientific and statistical inference.* Basingstoke, UK: Palgrave Macmillan.

Doya, K., Ishii, S., Pouget, A., & Rao, R. (2007). *Bayesian brain: Probabilistic approaches to neural coding.* Cambridge, MA: MIT Press.

Duffy, K. R., & Hubel, D. H. (2007). Receptive field properties of neurons in the primary visual cortex under photopic and scotopic lighting conditions. *Vision Research, 47,* 2569–2574.

Ecker, A. S., Berens, P., Keliris, G. A., Bethge, M., Logothetis, N. K., & Tolias, A. S. (2010). Decorrelated neuronal firing in cortical microcircuits. *Science, 327,* 584–587.

Einstein, A. (1920). *Relativity: The special and the general theory; A popular exposition* (R. W. Lawson, Trans.). London: Methuen.

Esch, H. E., Zhang, S., Srinivasan, M. V., & Tautz, J. (2001). Honeybee dances communicate distances measured by optic flow. *Nature, 441,* 581–583.

Exner, S. (1894). *Entwurf zu einer physiologischen Erklärung der psychischen Erscheinungen von Dr. Sigmund Exner: I. Theil.* Leipzig: F. Deuticke.

Farah, M. J. (2000). *The cognitive neuroscience of vision.* Oxford: Blackwell.

Ferster, D., & Miller, K. (2000). Neural mechanisms of orientation selectivity in the visual cortex. *Annual Review of Neuroscience, 23,* 441–471.

Feynman, R., Leighton, R. & Sands, M. (1964). *The Feynman lectures on physics.* Reading, MA: Addison-Wesley.

Fischer, B. J., & Pena, J. L. (2011). Owl's behavior and neural representation predicted by Bayesian inference. *Nature Neuroscience, 14,* 1061–1066.

Foldiak, P. (1991). Learning invariance from transformation sequences. *Neural Computation, 3*(2), 194–200.

Foldiak, P., & Young, M. (1995). Sparse coding in the primate cortex. In M. A. Arbib (Ed.), *The handbook of brain theory and neural networks* (pp. 895–898). Cambridge, MA: MIT Press.

Frisby, J. P., & Stone, J. V. (2010). *Seeing: The computational approach to biological vision.* Cambridge, MA: MIT Press.

Friston, K. (2009). The free-energy principle: A rough guide to the brain? *Trends in Cognitive Sciences, 13*(7), 293–301.

Ganguli, D., & Simoncelli, E. P. (2010). Implicit encoding of prior probabilities in optimal neural populations. *Advances in Neural Information Processing Systems, 23,* 658–666.

Gauthier, J. L., Field, G. D., Sher, A., Greschner, M., Shlens, J., Litke, A. M., & Chichilnisky, E. J. (2009). Receptive fields in primate retina are coordinated to sample visual space more uniformly. *Public Library of Science Biology, 7*(4), e1000063.

Gawne, T. J. (2000). The simultaneous coding of orientation and contrast in the responses of v1 complex cells. *Experimental Brain Research, 133,* 293–302.

Gawne, T. J., & Richmond, B. J. (1993). How independent are the messages carried by adjacent inferior temporal cortical neurons? *Journal of Neuroscience, 13,* 2758–2771.

Girshick, A. R., Landy, M. S., & Simoncelli, E. P. (2011). Cardinal rules: Visual orientation perception reflects knowledge of environmental statistics. *Nature Neuroscience, 14*(7), 926–932.

Glennerster, A., Tcheang, L., Gilson, S. J., Fitzgibbon, A. W., & Parker, A. J. (2006). Humans ignore motion and stereo cues in favor of a fictional stable world. *Current Biology, 16,* 428–432.

Gregory, R. L. (1997a). *Eye and brain: The psychology of seeing.* 5th ed. Oxford: Oxford University Press.

Gregory, R. L. (1997b). Knowledge in perception and illusion. *Philosophical Transactions of the Royal Society of London. Series B, Biological Sciences, 352,* 1121–1128.

Gross, C. G. (1992). Representation of visual stimuli in inferior temporal cortex. *Philosophical Transactions of the Royal Society of London. Series B, Biological Sciences, 335,* 3–10.

Haigh, J. (2003). *Taking chances.* Oxford: Oxford University Press.

Hartline, H. K. (1949). Inhibition of activity of visual receptors by illuminating nearby retinal areas in the Limulus eye. *Federation Proceedings, 8*(1), 69.

Hartline, H. K. (1967). Visual receptors and retinal interaction. In K. Siegbahn et al. (Eds.), *Les Prix Nobel en 1967* (pp. 242–259). Stockholm: Norstedt & Söner, 1969.

Hartline, H. K., & Graham, C. H. (1932). Nerve impulses from single receptors in the eye. *Journal of Cellular and Comparative Physiology, 1*(2), 277–295.

Hartline, H. K., & Ratliff, F. (1958). Spatial summation of inhibitory influences in the eye of Limulus, and the mutual interaction of receptor units. *Journal of General Physiology, 41,* 1049–1066.

Heeger, D. J. (1991). Nonlinear model of neural responses in cat visual cortex. In M. S. Landy & J. A. Movshon (Eds.), *Computational models of visual processing* (pp. 119–133). Cambridge, MA: MIT Press.

Heeger, D. J., Simoncelli, E. P., & Movshon, J. A. (1996). Computational models of cortical visual processing. *Proceedings of the National Academy of Sciences of the United States of America, 93,* 623–627.

Helmholtz, H., von (1867). *Handbuch der physiologischen Optik.* Leipzig: Voss.

Hirsch, J. A., Alonso, J. M., Reid, R. C., & Martinez, L. M. (1998). Synaptic integration in striate cortical simple cells. *Journal of Neuroscience, 18*(22), 9517–9528.

Hubel, D. (1988). *Eye, brain, and vision.* New York: W. H. Freeman.

Hubel, D., & Wiesel, T. N. (1979). Brain mechanisms of vision. In D. Flanagan et al. (Eds.), *The brain* (pp. 84–96). San Francisco: W. H. Freeman.

James, H. (1890). The principles of psychology. Reprinted 1950. New York: Dover.

Jaynes, E. T., & Bretthorst, G. L. (2003). *Probability theory: The logic of science: Principles and elementary applications* (Vol. 1). Cambridge: Cambridge University Press.

Johansson, G. (1973). Visual perception of biological motion and a model for its analysis. *Perception and Psychophysics, 14*, 201–211.

Jones, M. & Love, B. C. (2011). Bayesian fundamentalism or enlightenment? On the explanatory status and theoretical contributions of Bayesian models of cognition. *Behavioral and Brain Sciences, 34*, 169–188

Kaplan, E. (2003). The M, P, and K pathways of the primate visual system. In L. M. Chalupa & J. S. Werner (Eds.), *The visual neurosciences* (Vol. 1, pp. 481–493). Cambridge, MA: MIT Press.

Kersten, D., Mamassian, P., & Yuille, A. (2004). Object perception as Bayesian inference. *Annual Review of Psychology, 55*(1), 271–304.

Kersten, D., & Yuille, A. (2003). Bayesian models of object perception. *Current Opinion in Neurobiology, 13*, 150–158.

Knill, D. C. (2007a). Learning Bayesian priors for depth perception. *Journal of Vision, 7*(8), article 13.

Knill, D. C. (2007b). Robust cue integration: A Bayesian model and evidence from cue-conflict studies with stereoscopic and figure cues to slant. *Journal of Vision, 7*(7), article 5.

Knill, D. C., & Pouget, A. (2004). The Bayesian brain: The role of uncertainty in neural coding and computation. *Trends in Neurosciences, 27*(12), 712–719.

Knill, D. C., & Richards, R. (1996). *Perception as Bayesian inference.* New York: Cambridge University Press

Knill, D. C., & Saunders, J. A. (2003). Do humans optimally integrate stereo and texture information for judgments of surface slant? *Vision Research, 43*, 2539–2558.

Kording, K. P., & Wolpert, M. (2004). Bayesian integration in sensorimotor learning. *Nature, 427*, 240–247.

Kover, H. & Bao, S. (2010). Cortical plasticity as a mechanism for storing Bayesian priors in sensory perception. *PLoS ONE*, *5*(5), e10497, 05.

Kruppa, E. (1913).Zur ermittlung eines objecktes aus zwei perspektiven mit innerer orientierung. *Sitz.-Ber.Akad.Wiss., Math.Naturw., Kl.Abt.IIa*, *122*, 1939–1948.

Kuffler, S. W. (1953). Discharge patterns and functional organization of mammalian retina. *Journal of Neurophysiology*, *16*, 37–68.

Land, M. F., & Nilsson, D. E. (2002). *Animal eyes*. New York: Oxford University Press.

Laughlin, S. B. (1981). A simple coding procedure enhances a neuron's information capacity. *Zeitschrift für Naturforschung. Section C. Biosciences*, *36c*, 910–912.

Lee, D. N., & Aronson, E. (1974). Visual proprioceptive control of standing in human infants. *Perception & Psychophysics*, *15*(3), 529–532.

Lennie, P. (2003). The cost of cortical computation. *Current Biology*, *13*, 493–497.

Lettvin, J. Y., Maturana, H. R., McCulloch, W. S., & Pitts, W. H. (1959). What the frog's eye tells the frog's brain. *Proceedings of the Institute of Radio Engineers*, *49*, 1940–1951.

Lewis, A., & Zhaoping, L. (2006). Are cone sensitivities determined by natural color statistics? *Journal of Vision*, *6*(3), 285–302.

Logan, B. F., Jr. (1977). Information in the zero crossings of bandpass signals. *AT&T Technical Journal*, *56*, 487–510.

Logothetis, N. K., & Sheinberg, D. L. (1996). Visual object recognition. *Annual Review of Neuroscience*, *19*, 577–621.

Loh, A. (2006). The recovery of 3-D structure using visual texture patterns. Ph.D. thesis, University of Western Australia. Available at: http://en.scientificcommons.org/21371837]

Luria, A. R. (1976). *The working brain: An introduction to neuropsychology* (B. Haigh, Trans.). New York: Basic Books.

Machamer, P. K. (Ed.) (1998). *The Cambridge companion to Galileo*. Cambridge: Cambridge University Press.

MacLeod, D. I. A. (2003). New dimensions in color perception. *Trends in Cognitive Sciences*, *7*(3), 97–99.

Mallot, H. A. (2000). *Computational vision: Information processing in perception and visual behavior*. Cambridge, MA: MIT Press.

Marr, D. (1982). *Vision: A computational investigation into the human representation and processing of visual information*. Reprint, Cambridge, MA: MIT Press, 2010.

Marr, D., & Ullman, S. (1981). Directional selectivity and its use in early visual processing. *Proceedings of the Royal Society of London. Series B. Biological Sciences, 211*(1183), 151–180.

Martinez, L. M., Wang, Q., Reid, R. C., Pillai, C., Alonso, J. M. A., Sommer, F. T., et al. (2005). Receptive field structure varies with layer in the primary visual cortex. *Nature Neuroscience, 8*(3), 372–379.

Masland, R. H. (1969). Visual motion perception: Experimental modification. *Science, 165*, 819–821.

Mather, G., & Murdoch, K. (1994). Gender discrimination in biological motion displays based on dynamic cues. *Proceedings. Biological Sciences, 258*, 273–279.

McComb, D. M., Tricas, T. C., & Kajiura, S. M. (2009). Enhanced visual fields in hammerhead sharks. *Journal of Experimental Biology, 212*, 4010–4018.

McGrayne, S. B. (2011). *The theory that would not die: How Bayes' Rule cracked the Enigma Code, hunted down Russian submarines, and emerged triumphant from two centuries of controversy.* New Haven: Yale University Press.

McNeil, J. E., & Warrington, E. K. (1993). Prosopagnosia: A face-specific disorder. *Quarterly Journal of Experimental Psychology Section A, 46*(1), 1–10.

Meister, M., & Berry, M. J. (1999). The neural code of the retina. *Neuron, 22*, 435–450.

Mill, J. S. (1893). *A system of logic: Ratiocinative and inductive.* New York: Longmans, Green, and Co.

Miyashita, Y. (1988). Neuronal correlate of visual associative long-term memory in the primate temporal cortex. *Nature, 335*, 817–820.

Montgomery, G. (1995) How we see things that move. In M. Pines (Ed.), *Seeing, hearing, and smelling the world: New findings help scientists make sense of our senses* (pp. 24–30). Howard Hughes Medical Institute Report. Chevy Chase, MD: Howard Hughes Medical Institute.

Mountcastle, V. B. (1957). Modality and topographic properties of single neurons of cat's somatic sensory cortex. *Journal of Neurophysiology, 20*, 408–434.

Nadal, J. P., & Parga, N. (1993). Information processing by a perceptron in an unsupervised learning task. *Network* (Bristol, England), *4*(3), 295–312.

Nemenman, I., Lewen, G. D., Bialek, W., & de Ruyter van Steveninck, R. R. (2008). Neural coding of natural stimuli: Information at sub-millisecond resolution. *Public Library of Science Compututational Biology, 4*(3), e1000025, 03.

Neri, P. (2011). Coarse to fine dynamics of monocular and binocular processing in human pattern vision. *Proceedings of the National Academy of Sciences of the United States of America, 108*(26), 10726–10731.

Newton, I. (1704). *Opticks*. The Project Gutenberg EBook of Opticks. Available at http://www.gutenberg.org/files/33504/33504-h/33504-h.htm

Nilsson, D. E., & Pelger, S. (1994). A pessimistic estimate of the time required for an eye to evolve. *Proceedings. Biological Sciences, 256*(1345), 53–58.

Nirenberg, S., Carcieri, S. M., Jacobs, A. L., & Latham, P. E. (2001). Retinal ganglion cells act largely as independent encoders. *Nature, 411*(6838), 698–701.

Niven, J. E., Anderson, J. C., & Laughlin, S. B. (2007) Fly photoreceptors demonstrate energy-information trade-offs in neural coding. *Public Library of Science Biology, 5*(4), e116, 03.

Persi, E., Hansel, D., Nowak, L., Barone, P., & van Vreeswijk, C. (2011). Power-law input-output transfer functions explain the contrast-response and tuning properties of neurons in visual cortex. *Public Library of Science Computational Biology, 7*(2), e1001078, 02.

Pierce, J. R. (1980). *An introduction to information theory: Symbols, signals and noise.* 2nd ed. New York: Dover.

Purkinje, J. E. (1820). Beiträge zur näheren Kenntniss des Schwindels aus heautognostischen Daten. *Medicinische Jahrbücher des kaiserlich-königlichen österreichischen Staates, 6*, 79–125.

Purves, D., & Lotto, R. B. (2003). *Why we see what we do: An empirical theory of vision.* Sunderland, MA: Sinauer Associates.

Quiroga, R. Q., Reddy, L., Kreiman, G., Koch, C., & Fried, I. (2005). Invariant visual representation by single neurons in the human brain. *Nature, 435*(7045), 1102–1107.

Rao, R. P. N., & Ballard, D. H. (1999). Predictive coding in the visual cortex: a functional interpretation of some extra-classical receptive-field effects. *Nature Neuroscience, 2*, 79–87.

Regan, D. M. (2000). *Human perception of objects.* Sunderland, MA: Sinauer Associates.

Rescher, N. (1991). *G. W. Leibniz's "Monadology": An edition for students.* Pittsburgh: University of Pittsburgh Press.

Riddoch, G. (1917). Dissociation of visual perceptions due to occipital injuries, with especial reference to appreciation of movement. *Brain, 40*, 15–57.

Rieke, F., Warland, D., van Steveninck, R. R., & Bialek, W. (1997). *Spikes: Exploring the neural code.* Cambridge, MA: MIT Press.

Roorda, A. (2011). Adaptive optics for studying visual function: A comprehensive review. *Journal of Vision, 11*(5), article 6.

Rubens, A. B., & Benson, D. (1971). Associative visual agnosia. *Archives of Neurology*, *24*, 305–316.

Sacks, O., & Wasserman, R. (1996). *An anthropologist on Mars: Seven paradoxical tales*. New York: Vintage.

Salinas, E. (2011). Prior and prejudice. [this is a summary of papers by Girshick and Fischer listed here]. *Nature Neuroscience*, *14*, 943–945.

Salzman, C. D., Murasugi, C. M., Britten, K. H., & Newsome, W. T. (1992). Microstimulation in visual area MT: Effects on direction discrimination performance. *Journal of Neuroscience*, *12*(6), 2331–2355.

Saunders, P. T., Koeslag, J. H., & Wessels, J. A. (2000). Integral rein control in physiology ii. *Journal of Theoretical Biology*, *206*, 211–220.

Scholl, B. J. (2005). Innateness and (Bayesian) visual perception: Reconciling nativism and development. In P. Carruthers, S. Laurence, & S. Stich (Eds.), *The innate mind: Structure and contents* (pp. 34–52). Oxford: Oxford University Press.

Shannon, C. E. (1948). A mathematical theory of communication. *Bell System Technical Journal*, *27*, 379–423, 623–656.

Shannon, C. E., & Weaver, W. (1949). *The mathematical theory of communication*. Urbana: University of Illinois Press.

Simoncelli, E. (2003). Vision and the statistics of the visual environment. *Current Opinion in Neurobiology*, *13*(2): 144.

Simoncelli, E. P., & Olshausen, B. (2001). Natural image statistics and neural representation. *Annual Review of Neuroscience*, *24*, 1193–1216.

Sinha, P., & Poggio, T. (1996). Role of learning in three-dimensional form perception. *Nature*, *384*, 460.

Sobel, E. C. (1990). The locust's use of motion parallax to measure distance. *Journal of Comparative Physiology A: Neuroethology, Sensory, Neural, and Behavioral Physiology*, *167*, 579–588.

Srinivasan, M. V., Laughlin, S. B., & Dubs, A. (1982). Predictive coding: A fresh view of inhibition in the retina. *Proceedings of the Royal Society of London. Series B. Biological Sciences*, *216*(1205), 427–459.

Stocker, A. A., & Simoncelli, E. P. (2006). Sensory adaptation within a Bayesian framework for perception. *Advances in Neural Information Processing Systems Conference*, *18*, 1291–1298.

Stone, J. V. (1996). Learning perceptually salient visual parameters using spatiotemporal smoothness constraints. *Neural Computation*, *8*(7), 1463–1492.

Stone, J. V. (2001). Blind source separation using temporal predictability. *Neural Computation, 13*(7), 1559–1574.

Stone, J. V. (2004). *Independent component analysis: A tutorial introduction.* Cambridge, MA: MIT Press.

Stone, J. V. (2011). Footprints sticking out of the sand: 2. Children's Bayesian priors for lighting direction and convexity. *Perception, 4*(2), 175–190.

Stone, J. V., Kerrigan, I. S., & Porrill, J. (2009). Where is the light? Bayesian perceptual priors for lighting direction. *Proceedings. Biological Sciences, 276,* 1797–1804.

Stone, J. V., & Pascalis, O. (2010). Footprints sticking out of the sand: 1. Children's perception of naturalistic and embossed symbol stimuli. *Perception, 39,* 1254–1260.

Tanaka, K. (2004). Inferotemporal response properties. In L. M. Chalupa & J. S. Werner (Eds.), *The visual neurosciences* (Vol. 2, pp. 1151–1164). Cambridge, MA: MIT Press.

Thomas, R., Nardini, M., & Mareschal, D. (2010). Interactions between "light-from-above" and convexity priors in visual development. *Journal of Vision, 10*(8), article 6.

Todd, J. T. (1995). The visual perception of three-dimensional structure from motion. In W. Epstein & S. Rogers (Eds.), *Perception of space and motion* (pp. 201–226). 2nd ed. San Diego: Academic Press.

Tolhurst, D. J., & Dean, A. F. (1990). The effects of contrast on the linearity of spatial summation of simple cells in the cat's striate cortex. *Experimental Brain Research, 79*(3), 582–588.

Tootell, R. B., Switkes, E., Silverman, M. S., & Hamilton, S. L. (1988). Functional anatomy of macaque striate cortex: 2. Retinotopic organization. *Journal of Neuroscience, 8*(5), 1531–1568.

Ullman, S. (1979). *The interpretation of visual motion.* Cambridge, MA: MIT Press.

van der Willigen, R. F. (2011). Owls see in stereo much like humans do. *Journal of Vision, 11*(7), article 10.

van Hateren, J. H. (1992). A theory of maximizing sensory information. *Biological Cybernetics, 68,* 23–29.

Wang, G., Tanaka, K., & Tanifuji, M. (1996). Optical imaging of functional organization in the monkey inferotemporal cortex. *Science, 272,* 1665–1668.

Warren, W. H. (2004). Optic flow. In L. M. Chalupa & J. S. Werner (Eds.), *The visual neurosciences* (Vol. 2, 1247–1259). Cambridge, MA: MIT Press.

Wielaard, D. J., Shelley, M., McLaughlin, D., & Shapley, R. (2001). How simple cells are made in a nonlinear network model of the visual cortex. *Journal of the Neurological Sciences, 21*(14), 5203–5211.

Willshaw, D. J., & Buckingham, J. T. (1990). An assessment of Marr's theory of the hippocampus as a temporary memory store. *Philosophical Transactions of the Royal Society B, 329*, 205–215.]

Wiskott, L., & Sejnowski, T. (2002). Slow feature analysis: Unsupervised learning of invariances. *Neural Computation, 14*(4), 715–770.

Wohlgemuth, A. (1911). On the after-effect of seen movement. *British Journal of Psychology Monograph Supplements*, no. 1.

Yacoub, E. Harel, N., & Ugurbil K. (2008). High-field fMRI unveils orientation columns in humans. *Proceedings of the National Academy of Sciences, 105*(30), 10607–10612.

Zeki, S. (1993). *A vision of the brain.* Oxford: Blackwell.

Zhaoping, L. (Forthcoming). *Understanding vision: Theory, models, and data.* Online version available at http://www.cs.ucl.ac.uk/staff/Zhaoping.Li/prints/VisionTeach Book.pdf.

Zihl, J., von Cramon, D., & Mai, N. (1983). Selective disturbance of movement vision after bilateral brain damage. *Brain, 106*, 313–340.

Index